000125296863000
0123

MUCUSLESS DIET HEALING SYSTEM

A SCIENTIFIC METHOD OF EATING YOUR WAY TO HEALTH

PROF. ARNOLD EHRET

Introduction by
Dr. Benedict Lust

4,5612

4780612981 23

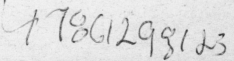

Beneficial Books are published by
BENEDICT LUST PUBLICATIONS
New York, New York 10156-0404 USA

Mucusless Diet Healing System
COPYRIGHT © 2002

Beneficial Books are published by

BENEDICT LUST PUBLICATIONS
New York, New York 10156-0404 USA

This Beneficial Book edition includes every word contained in Arnold Ehret's original book of 25 lessons for his students, plus new information from Dr. Benedict Lust's personal files. It is printed from brand new plates made from completely reset, clear, easy-to-read type.

Library of Congress Catalog Number 79-125412
ISBN 0-87904-004-1

Printed in the United States of America.

TABLE OF CONTENTS

reprinted from Dr. Benedict Lust's NATURO-PATH MAGAZINE

On October 8, 1922, Prof. Ehret held in Los Angeles, one of his most successful lectures. At least a hundred persons were unable to secure seats and had to be turned away (as Los Angeles laws allow no standing in aisles). Those of us who listened to his seemingly inspired and prophetic words will never forget the ardent, soul-stirring plea to humanity, made with all the forcefulness he could command, and expressing his unselfish devotion and keen desire to aid his suffering fellowmen.

Upon leaving the lecture hall, Prof. Ehret was hastily making his way to the railroad station to board the train for his home in the Los Angeles suburbs. He was wearing a pair of new shoes for the first time. The street was poorly lighted. In stepping off the curb, he lost his balance, falling backward and striking his head on the stone curbing. A few minutes after the fall he breathed his last, never regaining consciousness. The autopsy revealed a basal fracture of the skull.

Thousands of people, scattered in almost every part of the civilized world now mourn the loss of their teacher and friend. Tears that were shed were genuine and sincere, for he had endeared himself to a host of friends.

BIOGRAPHY OF ARNOLD EHRET

I knew Prof. Ehret first as an author, later as a sanitarium proprietor and lecturer, and now esteem him highly as a friend and a pioneer of the most complete, natural, and scientific system or cult for the Cure and Prevention of Disease known. I have no hesitancy in stating that he has evolved and developed what now seems to be the "last word" in regard to health and longevity.

Arnold Ehret was born near Freiburg, in Baden, Germany and was endowed by his father with a natural bent or extraordinary desire for delving into the causes and reasons for occurrences and results. His father bequeathed him a fine reputation of skill in treating animals as well as men without drugs and with natural remedies, with what seemed as "miraculous" success.

His education was obtained at a college where the long walk added to the work on the farm, on almost an ordinary vegetarian diet, brought on a severe attack of bronchial catarrh, but in spite of this, graduated with honor. His greatest interest being for physics, chemistry, drawing and painting, he took a special academy course and graduated as professor of drawing for high schools and colleges, at 21 years of age. He taught at a college until drafted for military service, but was released after nine month's service because of "neurasthenic heart trouble," resuming his vocation as a teacher. At 31 years of age was quite fleshy and looked well, as others said, but was suffering from kidney trouble, Bright's disease, with consumptive tendency.

In his own words, "five times I took vacations to recuperate, but finally was pronounced "incurable" and resigned. Then for five years I "suffered much from many physicians" (24 in all) and part of this suffering was to pay the bills of about $6,000, but with the result pronounced "incurable." Physically and nearly mentally bankrupt, I thought of suicide, but accidentally heard of naturopathy and was treated at a Kneipp sanitarium three different times, getting some relief and a desire to live, but not cured. Was treated at five or six other Nature Cure sanitariums and tried all other methods known in Europe, expending more thousands, with the result not down sick, but not healthy, either. I learned something from the experiences, though; the main symptoms were mucus or pus and albumin in the urine and pain in the kidneys. The doctors, thinking a clear urine indicated health, tried to stop these eliminations with drugs and to replace the albumin by a meat, egg, and milk diet, but it only increased the disastrous results. I reasoned out from these methods what seemed like a *great light* on the subject; that the right diet should be free from mucus and albumin. My naturopathic treatment drew out some of the mucus by baths, exercise, etc., but fed it back by wrong diet.

I resolved to face what seemed a tragedy for me (and does now to most chronically sick persons after getting no relief from doctors), and try for myself that which I had learned from past experience; that wrong eating was the *cause* and right eating *might* be the cure. There was vegetarianism, fruit and nut diet, numerous food "cures" and a few hints that fasting would help. I went to Berlin to study vegetarianism, as there were over twenty vegetarian restaurants there at that time. My first observation was that vegetarians were not much more healthy than meat eaters, for many looked sickly and pale. With the starchy food and milk I grew slowly worse, but started a course of study at the University of medicine, physiology, and chemistry. I visited a school of naturopathy, learned something of mental healing, Christian Science, magnetic healing, etc., etc., all to *try* to find out the real and fundamental truths of perfect health. Was more or less disappointed and next went to Nice, in southern France, and tried a radical fruit diet with the exception of a pint of milk a day, thinking then that I needed the albumin. I made no special application of the fruit diet to my condition, as most others did not, and received but little benefit. Some days I felt well and on others felt very bad, so I soon went back home, returning to the so-called "good eating", as lived and suggested by well-meaning friends, relatives and physicians. I had learned something about fasting, but it was opposed by all friends and relatives, even my former naturopathic doctor told my sister that to a person with Bright's disease a few days' fast would prove fatal.

The next winter I went to Algiers, in northern Africa. The mild climate and the wonderful fruits improved my condition and gave me more faith in nature's methods and an understanding of them, and I gained courage to try short fasts to assist the cleansing properties of fruit and climate, with such results that one morning of a well feeling day I chanced to notice in my mirror that my face had taken on an entirely new look, that of a younger and a healthy looking person. But on the next bad feeling day the old and sickly looking face returned, yet it did not last long and these alternating changes in my face impressed me as a "revelation" from nature that I had found out her methods in part and was on the right track, and I resolved to study them more and live them closer in my future life.

An indescribable feeling never known before of better health, more vital energy, better efficiency, and more endurance and strength came to me and gave me great joy and happiness just to be alive. This was not only of the physical, but there was a great change in my mental ability to perceive, to remember, greater courage and hope, and above all an insight into the spiritual which became like a sunrise, throwing light upon all higher and spiritual problems. All my faculties were improved, far surpassing their best during my healthiest and best youth. My physical efficiency and endurance became wonderfully increased. I took a bicycle trip of about 800 miles, from Algiers to Tunis, accompanied by a friend bicyclist who lived on ordinary diet. I was never behind him but often ahead towards night when endurance became the test. Keep in mind that I was formerly a candidate for death, so declared by the doctors, but now jubilant that I could surpass the most efficient, and a constant joy and exhilaration from having escaped the "slaughter house" of mankind, called "Scientific Medical Clinics."

Arriving home again, I demonstrated my ability and endurance to perform the hardest farm labor and in tests of strength superior to those in good training on the ordinary diet, but being surrounded by friends and relatives who were living in the ordinary way and coming in contact with professional men who were excited by fear that my discoveries were of true principles and would eventually succeed and surpass those they were practicing. I gradually took up the ordinary diet. Fasting was then very unpopular and living in the family of my sister who threatened to prevent it should I attempt one, I could not take up again what I firmly believed and had proven by actual experience, that fasting (simply eating less) was Nature's Omnipotent method of cleansing the body from the effects of wrong and too much eating. I had also found it the "Master Key" to mental and spiritual unfoldment and evolution. I had not neglected the study of the scientific reasons *why* fruit and mucusless foods were so efficient, and had found that they developed during the process of digestion what was known as *Grape-Sugar*, and from what was termed carbohydrates by analysts. My experience, tests, and experiments as well as cures, all showed that grape-sugar of fruits was the essential material of human food, giving the highest efficiency and endurance, and at the same time was the best eliminator of debris and the most efficient healing agent known for the human body.

This was in direct contradiction of the nitrogenous-albumin theory of the doctors and scientists and also of the more modern theory of "mineral salts". In 1909 I wrote an article denouncing the Metabolic theory and in 1912 learned that Dr. Thomas Powell of Los Angeles had made the same discovery and was making remarkable cures by using foods containing what he called "Organic Carbon", which is the same food ingredients that develop into grape-sugar during digestion. With the embryo of these discoveries in mind and my experiences I left my friends and relatives, who would have shortened my life by their well-meaning kindness, and accompanied by a young man who was won by my experience to try with me experimental diet and fasting for his ailments, the principal one being stuttering, went to southern France. Here during several months of experiments I renewed my experiences in Africa and won a firmer belief than ever that fruit diet and fasting were nature's infallible factors for regaining and maintaining a superior health than is enjoyed by most of civilized mankind.

The results obtained were often called miraculous, but were only marvelous because of their rareness. The knowledge I had gained of the wonderful methods by which nature carried on the cleansing from the impurities from wrong food, and then the regenerating, repairing, and strengthening, by the *right* food, was the marvel, but not a miracle.

Especially important were the results on this comparatively young man—ten years younger than I. We made tests with all the general foods of civilization after cleansing fasts. Our now more sensitive organs revolted at once against their undesirable elements and especially against combinations, giving the most convincing evidence that modern cooking, with its mixtures, with but little knowledge of their qualities, was the fundamental cause of all diseases. It is impossible to know what food really is and its effects until the body has been cleansed by nature's own method, a fast. I have never known of such experiments ever being made by any one, and the facts gained have now been so abundantly proven during many years of the most searching and difficult practice that they have raised my knowledge above all doubts or arguments about the dietetic opinions of others.

To test our efficiency at exhaustive labor, we took a trip through northern Italy, walking for 56 hours continuously without sleep or rest or food, only drink. This after a seven day fast and then only one meal of two pounds of cherries. This was called by the professional minds that knew of it a most marvelous test, from their viewpoint. From what came the energy for this efficiency? From Nitrogen, Albumin, Organic salts, Fats, Vitamines, or from what? After a 16-hour walk I made a test of knee bendings and arm extendings, 360 times in a few minutes, and later numerous strength tests with athletic competitors, showing superior results. These after being pronounced incurable and my father and brother having died of consumption. During our trip through Italy we were often the subjects of interesting comments by ladies on our ruddy and healthy complexion and inquiries of how we brought it about, etc. As a completely transformed man, I desired higher experiences, as they were not only physical, but mental and spiritual. The same with my young companion. He was wonderfully improved in many ways, but his stuttering showed no change. I had the idea that even that was caused by a physical encumbrance of debris. We proceeded to a secluded place on the island of Capri and there took longer fasts and daily sunbaths with heat around 120° of four to six hours. We were so well cleansed that we did not sweat. On the 18th day my young friend became quite hoarse, and fearing he would lose his voice— not then knowing what caused it—ended his fast with about three pounds of figs, at my suggestion, with the result that for nearly an hour he raised a very large quantity of mucus from his throat and his body cleansed itself in other directions. His voice soon being restored and his stuttering disappeared and has never returned. We had accomplished what his rich father had in vain tried to do by employing almost every known treatment for him, without the slightest permanent improvement.

Fasting, Nature's Supreme Remedy, has been so crudely practiced, and is so generally misunderstood that it is *very* important that it be rightly explained. From my long experience in curing myself by fasting and mucusless diet, and in conducting fasts for many hundreds in my sanitarium in Switzerland, during a period of over 10 years, I can state with certainty of its wonderful potency and benefits when rightly conducted. My first experiences brought such beneficial results that I desired to perfect and verify the methods employed, so I continued my observations and investigations of and into all phases of life. I made many and very extensive experiments, and then my fully restored young friend and myself started on a long producing power, and also a superior cleansing power, when rightly used, and in connection with an intelligent abstinence from any food, for the prevention as well as curing of diseases of all kinds. That when used in accordance with the individual's encumbrance with disease debris—not germs—and his age, occupation, climate, season of the year, etc., that even the then so-called incurable diseases were helped in a uniform and orderly manner, and a cure certain, if not too much encumbered by habits and age. The *right* kinds and less food as a preparation for short or longer fasts as the condition indicated, gives the digestive organs a rest or "vacation" from over-work, and then the resuming of eating by a selection of the *right* kinds, (this being *very important*), brings wonderfully surprising and beneficial results. I fasted for 24 days with such marvelously pleasing results, not only to my physical condition, but to my mental and my aspirations spiritually, that my enthusiasm increased to tell my friends and others of my discoveries, experiences and conclusive results. I could not describe my feelings, but told them they must experience them for themselves, which some took up at once. I commenced my educational work by public fasts and lectures, fasting twice in large German cities, and twice in Switzerland. I was sealed in a room by Notaries of State, and strictly watched and controlled by physicians, and with no outside interference or communications. One fast of 21 days, one of 24, one of 32, one of 49 days in Cologne, all within a period of 14 months. Between these fasts, and after, my work was lecturing, giving tests of physical and mental efficiency, proving the value of what I had learned and experienced, and these forced me teaching and advising others, writing articles, and starting a Sanitarium in Switzerland, and advising by correspondence.

My first written article was after my forty-nine day fast in Cologne, and published in a Vegetarian Magazine, stating quite a new experience from fasting, diet and healing of disease, in fact, of life itself and its enjoyment and prolongation. It had a sensational and revolutionizing effect. It brought me letters of inquiry from all parts of the world, and in Europe particularly, health seekers, reformers and medical men were soon divided into opposers and enthusiastic followers. These writings brought on a scientific controversy or fight over the new principles I had brought to light, that in Europe the two opposing combinations were known as "Ehretists" and "Non-Ehretists."

The *truth* of the Ehretists was well described by a prominent editor and reformer as follows: "He (Ehret) did not invent or originate fasting, or the use of fruit or improved diet, for those are well known and used long ago as good factors of Naturopathy, but what he did do was to originate an entirely new system of combining them as a systematic Healing method, on a basis of perfect Nutrition and Fasting."

My mucus theory—afterwards a proven fact—as the fundamental cause of all diseases, was more and more recognized, and consequently my system of healing, too. It has stood the test and brought what one writer has expressed as "Enormous success," and today has a platform, that: *Natural Treatment and Diet is the Most Perfect* and *Suc-*

cessful system of healing known. It has automatically named itself, "Nutro-Therapy," and its resulting "cult" "Naturopathy." For over ten years I wrote articles for health journals, lectured in the large cities of Europe, discussing the merits of the system with medical men and professionals, and treating thousands of patients at my "Fruit and Fasting Sanitarium" and by correspondence, and without changing the fundamental principles, but strengthening them by a better knowledge of their details and how to apply them for best results. From all these was evolved what is now becoming well known in this country—the name, *"Mucusless Diet."* I came to this country just before the war to visit the Panama Exposition, and to examine the fruits raised here, and particularly of California, and my enforced remaining here by the war has seemed providencial in finding those here who had similar advances, discoveries and experiences, and we are now advocating and bringing to public knowledge the same principles that were so successful in Europe, in relieving suffering humanity and preventing disease, and developing an improved race of people that will not know what diseased conditions are, and bring about a better civilized humanity."

In editing Prof. Ehret's life-work items, I am pleased to add that the discoveries made here by Dr. Thomas Powell, which I assisted in developing and adding to, were intuitively surmised by Prof. Ehret, and afterwards found to be proven by his results, and later by reference to chemist Hensel's scientific analysis of foods, corroborated, are that fruits and vegetables have elements which are

xiii

superior to those in any other foods, for producing vital energy, both in amount and quality. These elements or ingredients are known as "organized carbon" and "grape sugar." Their presence in sufficient quantities refutes the now current idea that the organic, mineral or tissue salts are the energy elements. They exist only in infinitesimal amounts in all foods, and part of them are drugs. Neither are the number of calories ("heat units" by calorimeter tests), reasonable basis for selecting a proper diet. My over 40 years of observation, experiences and research have proven conclusively to me that fruits and vegetables have all the tissue salts needed, and that the presence of actually well known ingredients in sufficient quantity are the energy and life supporting ingredients which make them the superior of all other foods, when the debris (mucus) from the "Mucus-rich" foods is eliminated. Then the full beneficial effect of the "Mucusless Diet" can be enjoyed.

Prof. B.W. Child

the nearer he is to divinity." Goethe says—"Man is what he eats." The facts and the wisdom of great men prove that the care and worry and relentless struggle for daily bread are but the pursuit of a phantom. "The Follies of our Bodily support are the main and principal causes of all disease", is the title of a book written by a Swiss physician.

The struggle for existence is primarily the effort to acquire the means to live in luxury, that is, above all to eat well and copiously. The truth about right nourishment is a book of seven seals to the public and scholars. Most people, especially the poorer, are under the impression that they are underfed, as compared with the luxurious fare of the rich. The fear of hunger weighs upon modern mankind like a nightmare; the privation of a single meal already causes nervousness. This morbid error, this tragical ignorance, this fatal delusion, is engendered and supported by erroneous medical doctrines.

The attempt to place the people upon a right diet will be crowned with success only by giving the people the straight truth. Restriction in general is only possible if one knows how much or little is absolutely necessary, and what are really the best and most valuable foodstuffs. New thoughts and truths penetrate only when they are practically demonstrated in the extreme by individual leaders. The people will not turn toward a new goal until they see a champion swimming against the stream of the old, wrong doctrine.

Nobody will forego pleasure unless forced to do so; nobody will voluntarily forego certain foods as long as he considers them best, as long as he does not know that there is something better, something vastly superior, something infinitely more perfect. The purest, most perfect and at the same time most palatable food of humanity can only be the one which was determined for him biologically, that is, by the law of nature, in its natural form.

If the human being was the most perfect at creation, then his food at that time must have been the most perfect and most nutritious form of diet, and therefore all the concoctions emanating from the modern kitchen must perforce be regarded as inferior, and they represent a retrogression and degeneration of humanity.

On the other hand, a frugivorian diet, as described in Genesis, is the higher and superior form of diet for the human race. If, therefore, a right diet is to meet with success, it is first necessary to dispel the fear of undernourishment in the public mind. If a determined, general restriction, and partial or entire elimination of bread, meat, eggs, milk, etc., shall be effected, then it must be proved and demonstrated by individual examples that it is not only possible to exist by eating fruit, but also that this paradisical, natural diet of humanity was the most palatable and perfect, and therefore can serve as such today. It must be demonstrated that a handful of fruit contains more nourishing nutriment-matter than an entire modern dinner, consisting of half a dozen courses. The value of the ideal palatable food and all forms of nourishment must be demonstrated by fruitarians.

But where are the strict fruitarians? They exist

only in theory in civilized life. He could only keep to it strictly when living an out-door life separated from civilized surroundings. He lived thus for two years with a friend who lived the same. During that time he made the most wonderful tests, which are described in his book "Rational Fasting." *

One cannot live on a strict fruit-diet in civilized life because the senses are so highly developed as to render life quite unpleasant and unenjoyable when associated with so-called healthy people. One must live on the "Mucusless Diet" and bring his entire sensibility more nearly in accord with his associates. Paradise diet does not harmonize with the Sodoms of civilization, nor can one "come over" to a strict fruit diet except by a transition through the "Mucusless Diet." That has to be carefully and gradually acquired and individually instructed.

The universe is ruled by laws which never change, therefore, as fruit was the paradisical food of the most perfect and God-like beings, it is to-day the superior health-giving and Paradise diet.

*Rational Fasting, by Arnold Ehret. Available by mail from Benedict Lust Publications, P.O. Box 404, New York, NY 10156. Price $4.95 plus S/H.

General Introductory Principles

LESSON I

Every disease, no matter what name it is known by Medical Science, is

CONSTIPATION

A clogging up of the entire pipe system of the human body. Any special symptom is therefore merely an extraordinary local constipation by more accumulated mucus at this particular place. Special accumulation points are the tongue, the stomach and particularly the entire digestive tract. This last is the real and deeper cause of bowel constipation. The average person has as much as ten pounds of uneliminated feces in the bowels continually, poisoning the blood stream and the entire system. Think of it!

Every sick person has a more or less mucus-clogged system, such mucus being derived from undigested and uneliminated, unnatural food substances, accumulated from childhood on. Details regarding this fact may be learned by reading my *"Rational Fasting and Regeneration Diet."*

My *"Mucus Theory"* and *"Mucusless Diet Healing System"* stand unshaken; it has proven the most successful *"Compensation-Action"* so-called cure against every kind of disease. By its systematic application thousands of declared-incurable patients could be saved.

The *Mucusless Diet* consists of all kinds of raw

and cooked fruits, starchless vegetables, and cooked or raw, mostly green-leaf vegetables. The *Mucusless Diet Healing System* is a combination of individually advised long or short fasts, with progressively changing menus of *non-Mucus-Forming Foods. This Diet Alone Can Heal Every Case of "Disease"* without fasting, although such a cure requires longer time. The *System* itself will be expounded in later lessons.

However, to learn how to apply the system, to understand how and why it works, it is necessary to free your mind from Medical errors, partly taken over by Naturopathy. In other words, I must teach you a new Physiology, free from medical errors; a new method of *Diagnosis*; a correction of the Fundamental errors of *Metabolism*, high Protein foods, Blood circulation, Blood composition, and last, but not least, you must be taught

WHAT VITALITY REALLY IS

To Medical Science the Human body is still a mystery, especially in diseased condition. Every new disease "discovered" by the Doctors is a new mystery for them. There are no words to express how far they are away from the truth. Naturopathy uses the word *Vitality* continually. Yet neither "Medical Scientists" nor Naturopaths can tell what *Vitality* is.

Not only is it necessary to eradicate all these errors from your brain, but to show you the truth in such a new and simple light that you can grasp it at once. This great advantage of simplicity and clarity is one of the fundamental reasons for my success. Withal, my teachings cover the *Truth*. Incidentally, whatever *Simple Reason* cannot grasp is *Humbug*, however *Scientific* it may sound.

You will learn how wrong and ignorant it is to believe that any special disease can be healed by eating the right food, living upon "Special Menus" or undergoing long fasts, if such is done without experience and without system and special advice for each individual case.

"Fasting" has been known for hundreds of years as a "compensation" against every disease, as Nature's only and infallible law, and the same with the *Mucusless* diet, as already stated in Genesis (fruits and herbs, i.e. Green leaves). But why did it never come into general use and resultant universal success? Because it was never used systematically in accordance with the condition of the patient. The average man has not the slightest idea what the necessary eliminative process is; what time it requires; how and how often his diet must be changed; what it means to cleanse the body of the terrible quantities of waste he has accumulated in his body during his life.

Disease is an effort of the body to eliminate waste, mucus and toxemias, and this system assists nature in the most perfect and natural way. Not the disease but the body is to be healed, it must be cleansed, freed from waste and foreign matter, from mucus and toxemias accumulated since childhood. You cannot buy health in a bottle, you cannot heal your body, that is, cleanse your system in a few days, you must make "compensation" for the wrong you have done your body all during your life.

My system is not a cure or a remedy, it is a

regeneration, a thorough house-cleaning, the acquisition of such clean and perfect health as you never knew before.

Remember: Your constitutional encumbrances throughout the entire system are the source of every disease; the greatest and most harmful source of lowered vitality, imperfect health, lack of strength and endurance and any and all imperfect conditions. All have their source in the colon, never perfectly emptied since your birth. Nobody on earth today has an ideally clean body, and therefore perfectly clean blood. What Medical Science calls Normal health is in fact a pathological condition.

In Summa: The Human mechanism is an elastic pipe system . The Diet of Civilization is never entirely digested and the resultant waste eliminated. This entire pipe system is slowly constipated, especially at the place of the symptom and the digestive tract. This is the foundation of every disease. To loosen this waste, eliminate it intelligently and carefully, and to control this operation can only be done perfectly by the

MUCUSLESS-DIET HEALING SYSTEM

Latent, Acute and Chronic Diseases
No Longer a Mystery

LESSON II

The first lesson has now given you an insight as to what disease actually is. In addition to mucus and its toxemias in the system, there are other foreign matters such as uric acid, toxins, etc., and especially drugs if ever used. I learned thru years of practical experience that drugs are NEVER eliminated as is the waste from foods — but are stored up in the body for decades! Hundreds of cases have come under my observation where drugs taken 10, 20, 30 and even 40 years were expelled together with mucus thru this perfect healing system. *This is a fact of basic importance — especially for the Practitioner.* When these chemical poisons after being dissolved are taken back into circulation for elimination thru the kidneys — the nerves and heart are affected — causing extreme nervousness, dizziness and excessive heart-beats, as well as other strange sensations. The uninformed stands before a mystery and probably calls the family doctor, who now diagnoses the condition as "heart-disease" and blames the "lack of food" instead of the drugs he prescribed 10 years ago.

The average "normal" man, considered healthy, has a chronic, stored-up accumulation of waste food — poisons and drugs.

THIS IS HIS LATENT DISEASE

When these latent disease matters are occasionally stirred up, for instance by a cold, he expels great quantities of mucus, and feels unhappy instead of enjoying nature's cleansing process. If the quantity of loosened mucus is great enough to shock the entire system, more or less, but still not dangerous, it may be diagnosed as Influenza. If the eliminating work of nature digs deeper into the system, especially into that important organ — the lungs — so much mucus and poisons are loosened at once, that the circulation has to work under great friction, similar to a dirty machine — or, for example, an automobile running with its brakes set. The friction produces abnormal heat, which is called fever, and the doctors call it Pneumonia, which is really a "feverish" effort on nature's part to free the MOST VTAL organs from its waste. If the kidneys are called upon to eliminate this loosened mucus, thereby shocking this organ, it is called Nephritis, and etc.

In other words, whenever nature endeavors to save a human life thru her efforts to eliminate "feverishly" mucus and its toxic products, it is called:

ACUTE DISEASE

The Medical profession has over 4000 names for different ailments. The particular or special name of the disease is made up according to the respective local place of elimination; or to the congested point where the blood stream finds it difficult of passage and causes pain — such as pains in the joints, as in cases of rheumatism, for example.

For ages, this well-meaning effort and intended self-healing work of nature has been misunderstood and suppressed thru the agency of drugs, and the continuance of eating, despite the warning danger signals of pain and loss of appetite. Notwithstanding the "help" of the doctors — a help, in fact, injurious and dangerous to the patient's life — his vitality and especially his eliminating abilities are lowered, and nature proceeds slowly. Under this handicap nature cannot work as efficiently, requiring more time, and the case is called "Chronic." The word chronic is derived from the Greek word "chronos," meaning time. You will be taught in Lesson 7 more about this mystery.

The Diagnosis

LESSON III

WHY THE DIAGNOSIS?

Laymen and even some dietetic experts with the exception of myself, believe there is no need for diagnosis. You may ask, since there is only one disease why the diagnosis? If all sickness is due to uncleanliness from uneliminated, undigested food, mucus, uric acid, toxemias, drugs, etc., why diagnose? We shall now learn why fruit-diet and fasting have produced such doubtful results, thru their incorrect use and misunderstanding, caused thru the belief that general rules of this cure are suitable for everybody and for every case. Nothing is further from the truth! No other cure requires so much individual specialization and continual changing to meet the reaction of the patient. This is why people who attempt these methods of cure without expert advice frequently bring about serious results.

PROMISCUOUS FASTING

McFadden, and many others, advise, for instance, fasting as applicable to all cases. I learned thru thousands of cases during my experience that nothing requires more individual, different application than fasting and the mucus-less diet. Of two patients — one may effect a complete recovery after a fast of two or three weeks, while the other *may die from the same treatment!* That is why an individual diagnosis of general conditions and constitutional encumbrances is so necessary.

METHOD OF CONSTITUTIONAL DIAGNOSIS

My diagnosis determines the following points:

1. The relative amount of encumbrance in the system.

2. The predominant part, that is, whether more mucus or more poisons.

3. If pus is present in the system, amount and kind of drugs used.

4. If internal tissue or an organ is in a process of decomposition.

5. How far vitality is lowered.

You will also learn thru experience and observations along these lines that the general appearance, especially the face of the patient, will indicate more or less the internal conditions.*

MEDICAL DIAGNOSIS

Medical diagnosis throws no real light on the subject, although doctors think it more important than the actual cure. It is made up of a series of reports of symptoms and a scheme of experiences from which thousands of diseases are named. Characteristic of the meaningless medical diagnosis is the frequent statement of many patients that "the doctors could not find out what I have." THE NAME OF THE DISEASE DOES NOT CONCERN US AT ALL. A man with gout, one with indigestion, or one with Bright's disease may start with the same advice. Whether to fast, for instance, and how long, does not depend

*For further information refer to "The Magic Mirror," page 18.

upon the name of the disease, but upon the patient's condition and how far vitality is lowered.

NATUROPATHIC CONCEPTS

Naturopathy is an advance over medicine in teaching that all disease is constitutional. Naturopathy does not explain sufficiently the source, nature and composition of "foreign matters" as the fundamental one-ness of all disease.

Dr. Lahmann said: "Every disease is caused by carbonic acid and gas." But he did not learn its source in decayed, uneliminated food substance — the mucus in a state of continuous fermentation.

Dr. Jaeger said: "Disease is a stench." Nature gives a diagnose thru bad odor, which indicates how far the inside decomposition has progressed.

Dr. Haigh of England, the founder of the "Anti-uric-acid diet," bases his conception of general diagnose on the asumption that the majority of diseases are caused thru uric acid, certainly an important part of diseased matter besides mucus.

URIC DIAGNOSIS

Medical doctors and many others consider this special kind of diagnosis as the most important one, but it is fundamentally misunderstood. Besides the digestive tract, the uric canal is the main avenue of elimination. *As soon as any one decreases his eating, fasts a little, or changes over to the natural diet, he has waste, mucus, poisons, uric acid, phosphates, etc., in his urine,* and an analysis of his urine is alarming. This same thing happens in the majority

of cases whenever any one becomes sick. Every one
becomes alarmed at this effort of the body to eliminate waste — which is in truth the healing, cleansing process.

Should sugar or albumen be found in the urine
the case is called "very serious," and diagnosed
"Diabetes," or "Bright's disease," respectively. Under medical treatment the patient in the first named
case, dies thru sugar-starvation, caused thru lack
of sugar and sugar-formers in the dietary. In the
latter diagnosis the patient dies from forced "albumen replacement" resulting from over-feeding of
foods rich in albumen.

WHATEVER THE BODY EXPELS IS WASTE, DECAYED,
DEAD — and simply indicates that the patient is in
an advanced state of inside uncleanliness, already
causing a decomposition of inside organs — producing rapid decay of all food taken into the body.
These cases — like tuberculosis, must be treated
very carefully and *VERY SLOWLY*.

HOW IT LOOKS IN THE HUMAN COLON

It is of utmost importance that thru our diagnose
we must learn as much as possible the general
appearance of the inside of the human body. Our
diagnosis therefore consists in finding out the degree
of quantities of individual waste matter of the
patient.

Experts in autopsy state they have found that
from 60 to 70% of the colons examined have foreign
matters such as worms and decades old feces-stones.
The inside walls of the over-intestines are encrusted

by old, hardened feces and resemble in appearance the inside of a filthy stove-pipe.

I had fat patients that eliminated from their body as much as 50 to 60 pounds waste, and 10 to 15 pounds alone, from the colon — mainly consisting of foreign matters, especially old, hardened, feces. The average so-called "healthy" man of today carries continually with him, since childhood, several pounds of never-eliminated feces. One "good stool" a day means nothing. A fat and sick man is in fact a living "cess-pool." A distinct surprise to me was that a number of my patients in such condition had already undertaken *so-called* "nature cures."

Diagnosis — (Continued)

LESSON IV

FAT AND LEAN TYPES

The bodily mechanism of the fat type is, on the average, *mechanically* more obstructed, because he is in general an over-eater of starchy foods. In the lean type there is more *physiological* chemical interference with the organism, such a one being in general a one-sided meat eater, which condition produces especially, much acidity, uric acid, other poisons and pus.

DISEASE STORY

As a general rule I ask my prospective patients the following questions as the knowledge to be gained is of great importance:
1. How long have you been sick?
2. What did the doctor call your disease?
3. What was the nature of the treatment?
4. How much and what kinds of treatment taken?
5. Have you ever been operated upon?
6. What other kinds of treatment have you taken before?

(Age, sex, whether a disease is inherited, etc., are important points.)

The most important thing, however, is the patient's diet at present, his special craving for certain foods and his wrong habits; if constipated, and how long. What kind of diets, if any, were used before. It is necessary to base the change in diet on the patient's present diet, and only A SLIGHT CHANGE toward an improved diet is advisable.

THE EXPERIMENTAL DIAGNOSIS

THE MOST EXACT, UNERRING DIAGNOSIS WE HAVE IS A SHORT FAST. The more rapidly the patient feels "worse" thru a short fast, the greater and the more poisonous is his encumbrance. Should he become dizzy, suffer severe headaches, etc., he is greatly clogged up with mucus and toxemias. If palpitation of the heart occurs *it is a sign that pus is somewhere in the system*, or that drugs, even though taken many years ago, are in the circulation for elimination.

Any inside special "constipated" place is located by a light pain there. The experimental practitioner can ascertain better than with X-rays through nature's revelation after a short fast the true condition of the inside of the human body, and knows the real diganosis more correctly than doctors can ascertain with all their expensive scientific equipment and instruments.

If this "short-fast" diagnosis is tried on the average man called normal and healthy — but in reality clogged up with mucus — latent disease — nature reveals the same to you in a moderate degree, and if a "weak point" has begun to develop, unsuspected by them, nature will unerringly indicate where and how he will later become sick if the wrong method of living is continued, although it may be after some years. This then is the PROGNOSIS OF DISEASE.

SOME SPECIAL DIAGNOSIS

To show that all differently named diseases, even the most severe ones, have their basis and are caused by the same general and constitutional encumbrance of the body, I shall show you, in the light of truth, a few characteristic kinds of cases. Thru these *illustrative examples* I shall prove that there is not a single disease, not a disturbance or sensation, not an unhealthy appearance or symptom, which cannot be explained and seen at once in its real nature as local constipation, constitutional constipation, by mucus and its toxemias; most of the quantities continually supplied from the "chronic reserve stock of waste" in the stomach, intestines, and especially, in the colon. The "basement" of the human "temple" is the reservoir from which every symptom of disease and weakness is supplied in all its manifestations.

A Cold

Is a beneficial effort to eliminate waste from the cavities of the head, the throat and the bronchial tubes.

Pneumonia

The cold goes deeper and will eliminate and clean the mucus from the most spongy and vital organ, the lung. A hemorrhage occurs to clean more radically. The entire system is aroused, causing higher temperature by friction of the waste in circulation. That proves alarming, and the doctor suppresses by drugs and food, actually blocking nature's process of healing — cleansing. If the patient does not die, the elimination becomes chronic and is called

CONSUMPTION

The consumptive patient eliminates continually his mucus caused from erroneously increased, mucus-forming foods, thru the lungs instead of thru the natural ways. This organ itself decays more and more, producing germs, and it is then called tuberculosis.

The vital organ (lung) — the pump — works insufficiently on the circulation, the entire cell system decays more and more, and decomposes before the patient dies.

TOOTHACHE

Its pain is a warning signal of nature; "stop eating; I must repair; there is waste and pus; you have eaten too much lime-poor food, meat."

RHEUMATISM AND GOUT

Mucus and uric acid particularly accumulated in the joints, since here is the less dependable part of the tissues for the passage of the circulation, heavily loaded with waste and uric acid in the one-sided meat eater's body.

The stomach is the central organ of disease matter supply. There is a limit to the ability of this organ to digest and to empty itself after the meal. Every food (even the best kinds) are mixed with this acid mucus, continually remaining in the average person's stomach. The wonder is how long the human being can stand such conditions.

GOITER

is a deposit by nature of tremendous waste to keep it from entering the circulation.

A Boil
is in principle the same, only the elimination is outside.

Stammering
Special accumulation of mucus in the throat, in-
terfering with the functioning of the vocal chords.
I cured several cases.

Liver and Kidney Diseases
These organs are of a very spongy construction,
and their function is that of a kind of physiological
sieve. They are, therefore, easily constipated by
sticky mucus.

Sex Diseases
These have for their origin nothing more than
mucus elimination thru these organs, and are easily
healed. The use of drugs alone produces the characteristic symptoms of syphilis. The more drugs
that have been used, especially mercury, the more
carefully the treatment must be conducted.

Ear and Eye Diseases
Even short or long sight is congestion in the eyes
and trouble with hearing congestion of those organs.
I healed a few kinds of blindness and deafness by
the same principles.

MENTAL DISEASES

Besides a congested system, I found that any one
mentally diseased has congestion, especially of the
brain. One man on the verge of insanity was cured
by a four weeks' fast. There is nothing easier to heal
than insanity by fasting — such men having lost

their reason, their natural instinct tells them not to eat. I learned that if you heal by the Mucusless-diet Healing System all kinds of diseases, most of the patients are relieved of greater or less mental conditions. After a fast comes a clearer mind. Unity of ideas comes to take the place of differences. Differences of ideas today are caused largely by diet. If something is wrong with any one, look first to the stomach. The mentally diseased man suffers physiologically from gas pressure on the brain.

The Magic Mirror
SUPPLEMENT TO DIAGNOSIS
LESSONS III AND IV

Since man degenerated thru civilization, he no longer knows what to do when he becomes sick. Disease remains the same mystery to modern medical science as it was to the "Medicine Man" of thousands of years ago—the main difference being that the "germ" theory has replaced the "Demon" and that mysterious, outside power remains—to harm you and destroy your life.

Disease is a mystery to you as well as to every doctor who has not as yet looked into the "magic mirror" which I am about to explain. Naturopathy deserves full credit for having proven that disease is within you—a foreign matter which has weight—and which must be eliminated.

If you want to become your own physician, or, if you are a Drugless Healer and want more success, you must learn the truth and know what disease is. You cannot heal yourself, or other people, without an exact diagnosis which will give you a clear idea of true conditions. This infallible truth can be learned only from the book of Nature—that is: Thru a test on your own body—or the "magic mirror," as I have designated it.

The sufferer from any kind of disease—or any person, whether sick or not—will go thru this healing process of fasting and mucusless diet, will eliminate mucus—thereby demonstrating that the basic cause of all latent diseases of man is a clogged-up tissue system of un-eliminated, un-used and undigested food substances.

Thru the "magic mirror" a true and unfailing diagnosis of your disease is furnished, as never before.

"THE MAGIC MIRROR"

1. Proof that your personal, individual symptom, sore, or sensation, according to what your disease is named, is nothing more than an extraordinary *local accumulation of waste*.

2. The coated tongue is evidence of a constitutional encumbrance thruout the entire system, which obstructs and congests the circulation by dissolved mucus, and this mucus even appears in the urine.

3. The presence of unevacuated feces, retained thru sticky mucus in the pockets of the intestines, constantly poisoning, and thereby interfering with proper digestion and blood-building.

To look inside your body—far better and clearer than can be done by doctors with expensive X-ray apparatus—and learn the cause of your disease, or even discover some hitherto unknown physical imperfection or mental condition, try this:

Fast one or two days, or eat fruits only (such as oranges, apples, or any juicy fruit in season) for two or three days, and you will notice that your tongue will become heavily coated. When this happens to the acutely sick, the doctor's conclusion is always—"indigestion." The tongue is the mirror not only of the stomach, but of the entire membrane system, as well. The fact that this heavy coating returns, even if removed by a tongue scraper once or twice a day, is an accurate indication of the amount of filth, mucus and other poisons accumulated in the tissues of your entire system, now being eliminated on the inside surface of the stomach, intestines and every cavity of your body.

After you have fasted, it is advisable to decrease the quantity of your customary amount of food—and eat only natural, cleansing, mucusless foods (fruits and starchless vegetables) thereby affording the body an opportunity to loosen and eliminate mucus, which is, in fact, THE HEALING PROCESS.

This "mirror" on the tongue's surface reveals to the observer the amount of encumbrance that has been clogging up the system since childhood—thru wrong, mucus-forming foods. After observing the urine during this test, by allowing it to stand for a few hours, you will note the elimination of quantities of mucus in same.

The actual amount of filth and waste, which is the "mysterious" cause of your "trouble," is almost unbelievable.

Disease—every disease—is, first: A special, local

constipation of the circulation; tissues; pipe system. The manifestation of symptoms, or, of the different symptoms. If painful and inflamed, it is from over-pressure—heat or inflammation caused by friction and congestion.

Second: Disease—every disease—is constitutional constipation. The entire human pipe system, especially the microscopically small capillaries are "chronically" constipated, through the wrong food of civilization.

White blood corpuscles are waste—and there is no man in Western civilization who has mucus-free blood and mucus-free blood vessels. It is like the soot in a stove-pipe which has never been cleaned; in fact, worse—because the waste from protein and starchy foods is STICKY.

The characteristics of tissue construction, especially of the important internal organs, such as the lungs, kidneys, all glands, etc., are very much similar to those of a sponge. *Imagine a sponge soaked in paste or glue!*

Naturopathy must more and more, cleanse its science from medical superstitions—wrongly called "scientific diagnosis." Nature, alone, is the teacher of a standard science of truth. She heals thru one thing—FASTING—every disease that it is possible to heal. This, alone, is proof that Nature recognizes but one disease, and that in every body the largest factors are always, waste, foreign matter and mucus (besides uric acid and other toxemias, and, very often, pus—if tissues are decomposed).

In order to realize how terribly clogged up the human body is, one must have seen thousands of fasters—as I have. The almost inconceivable fact is: How can such quantities of waste be stored up in the body? Have you ever stopped to realize the masses of phlegm you expel during a cold? And just as it is taking place in your head—your bronchial tubes, lungs, stomach, kidneys, bladder, etc., have the same appearance. All are in the same condition. And the spongy organ known as the tongue accurately mirrors on its surface the appearance of every other part of your body.

Medicine has devised a "special science" of laboratory tests, urinal diagnosis and blood tests.

More than fifty years ago, the most prominent pioneers of Naturopathy said: "Every disease is foreign matter—waste." I said, twenty years ago, and repeat it again and again, that most of these foreign matters are paste produced from wrong foods, decomposed—to be seen when it leaves the body as mucus. Meat decomposes into pus.

The light of truth dawned upon me after I had fasted, against the will of the Naturopath from whom I was taking treatments for Bright's disease. When the test-tube filled up with albumen, I read his thoughts in his facial expression. But to me it proved that whatever Nature expels—eliminates— is waste; whether it be albumen, sugar, mineral salts or uric acid. This occurred more than twenty-four years ago, but this Nature-doctor (a former M.D.) still believes in the replacement of albumen by high protein foods.

The medical diagnosis of Bright's Disease, when the chemical test of urine shows a high percentage of albumen, is as misleading as others. The elimination of albumen proves that the body does not need it, that it is over-fed—over-loaded with high protein stuff. Instead of decreasing these poison-producing foods, they are wrongly increased—endeavoring to replace the "loss"—until the patient dies. How tragic to replace waste, while Nature is endeavoring to save you, by removing it!

The next important laboratory test is that of sugar in the urine—Diabetes. The medical dictionary still calls it "mysterious." Instead of eating natural sweets, which go into the blood, and which can be used—the diabetic patient is fed eggs, meat, bacon, etc., and, in fact, actually starves to death thru lack of natural, sugar-containing and sugar-producing foods, which have been withheld.

It has long since been proven that all of these blood tests, especially the Wasserman test, are a fallacy.

We, as Naturopaths, cannot ignore Nature's teaching, in any way; even tho we may find it difficult to discard old errors hammered into us since childhood.

One of the most misleading errors is the individual naming of all diseases. The name of any disease is not important, and not of any value, whatsoever, when starting a natural cure—especially thru fasting and diet. If every disease is caused thru foreign matters—and it most assuredly is—then it is only important and necessary to know, how great and how much the amount of the patient's encumbrance actually is—how far and how much his system is clogged up by foreign matters, and how much his vitality has become lowered (See Lesson 5), and, in case of tuberculosis or cancer, if the tissues, themselves, are decomposed. (Pus and germs.)

I have had hundreds of cases tell me that every

doctor they called upon gave a different diagnosis, and a correspondingly different name for their ailment. I always surpise them by saying: "I know exactly what ails you—thru facial diagnosis—and you will see it, yourself, in the 'magic mirror,' within a few days."

THE EXPERIMENTAL DIAGNOSIS

Just as I have already stated in the beginning of this lesson, you must fast for two or three days. In the case of a fatty type, liquids should be used during the fast. The surface of the tongue will clearly indicate the appearance on the inside of the body, and the patient's breath will prove the amount and grade of decomposition. It is even possible to tell the kind of food they preferred most!

Should pain be felt at any one place, during the beginning of the fast, you may be sure that this is a weak point—and the symptom is not sufficiently developed for medical doctors to reveal it, thru their examination.

Waste will show up in the urine with clouds of mucus, and mucus will be expelled from the nose, throat and lungs as well as in the faeces. The weaker and more miserable the patient may feel during the fast, the greater is his encumbrance, and the weaker his vitality.

This experimental diagnosis tells you exactly what the trouble is, and how to correct it by starting with a moderate transition diet—or a more radical one—and whether to continue or discontinue the fast.

This experiment is the foundation—the basis of

the development of the science of Nature cure, physics, chemistry, etc. It is the question put to Nature, and she replies with the same infallible answer, always and everywhere.

If a patient becomes nervous, or symptoms of heart trouble occur, you may be sure that he has drugs stored up in his body. A consumptive patient starts with such terrible elimination, after a short fast, that it must be plain to all how ignorant and how impossible it is to try and cure him with "good nourishing foods" such as eggs and milk.

The above explanation is the experimental diagnosis, and the only scientific one. You cannot secure a better view inside than by this simple method. No expensive apparatus can show more accurately the exact conditions as they exist inside the body. All other examinations, including iris-diagnosis, diagnosis of the spine, etc., are never exact, and, therefore, not dependable.

Nature's mirrors; her revelations; her demonstrations—of and by phenomena—are "magic" only so long as you lack the correct interpretation of them. Nature shows and plainly reveals to you, everything—far more exact, perfect and better than all "science of diagnosis," put together.

THE PROGNOSIS OF DISEASE

And now we come to the prognosis of disease. We hear of "latent" disease. Every one, no matter to what extent he may enjoy "good health," has a latent sickness—and Nature only awaits an opportunity to eliminate the waste stored up since childhood—and on.

Everyone knows, but fails to understand, that a severe "shock," such as a cold—or "influenza" over the entire body, starts an elimination, but, unfortunately, Nature is handicapped in her attempted housecleaning, thru the doctor's advice to continue eating, thru the use of drugs, etc., *obstructing* elimination, and producing acute and chronic diseases.

Any one, even tho not sick—especially in the critical stage between thirty and forty—may fast a few days, and, thru the "magic mirror," learn the extent of his latent disease; where his weak point is located—as well as the name of his latent disease, and where it will appear. That is the prognosis of disease, and, if life insurance companies would only believe in it, would furnish a true and safe method of determining "risks."

Fasting until the tongue is clean is dangerous. Who can explain why the tongue becomes clean after breaking a short fast with a "square" meal, and why the "magic mirror" shows up more waste, if you live on fruits or mucusless diet, after the fast? This is the hitherto unexplained mystery of the "Magic Mirror." And the simple explanation is: That the elimination is *stopped* for a while, thru the eating of wrong foods—and as a result you feel better for a time, with wrong foods, than with fruits. And during this period even the "Magic Mirror" apparently leads you into thinking the body is clean. A return to natural foods soon proves otherwise.

For the ordinary person, it will require from one to three years of systematically continued fastings, and natural, cleansing diet, before the body is *actually cleansed of* "foreign matters." You may then see how the body is constantly eliminating waste, thru the entire outside surface of the body, from every pore of the skin; the urinal canal, and the colon; from the eyes and ears; and from the nose and throat. You can see how wet as well as dry mucus (dandruff, for instance), is being expelled. All diseases, therefore, are immense quantities of waste, "chronically" stored up, and thru this artificial elimination of "chronic disease" you will agree with me, and realize that I am not exaggerating when I state:

The diagnosis of your disease—of all diseases of mankind, both mental and physical, since the beginning of civilization, proves that they all have the same foundational cause—whatever the symptoms be. It is, without exception, one and the same general and universal condition—a one-ness of all disease, that is: Waste, foreign matter, mucus and its poisons.

"Internal impurity" is too mild an expression for chronic constipation. Waste—filth—mucus—stench (offensive odor) or "Invisible Waste," is the true description.

The Formula of Life
The Secret of Vitality

LESSON V

'V' = 'P' - 'O' ('V' equals 'P' minus 'O') *is the formula of Life*—and yet at the same time you may call it the formula of death.

"V" stands for VITALITY.

"P" or call it "X" the unknown quantity in this question, is the POWER that drives the human machinery, which keeps you alive, which gives you strength and efficiency—endurance for as yet an unknown length of time without food!

"O" means OBSTRUCTION, encumbrance, foreign matter, toxemias, mucus—in short, all internal impurities which obstruct the circulation, the function of internal organs especially; and the human engine in its entire functioning system.

You can therefore see thru this equation that as soon as "O" becomes greater than "P" the human machine must come to a standstill.

The Engineer can figure exactly "E = P - F"; meaning that the amount of energy or efficiency "E" he secures from an engine is not equal to the power "P" without first deducting "F," the friction.

The ingenious idea of construction of the ideal engine is to make it work with the smallest amount of friction. Should we transfer this fundamental and principal idea on the human engine, we see that it involves the terrible ignorance of medical physiology and that naturopathy found a true way of healing by removing—eliminating obstructions—that is, foreign matters of encumbrance, mucus and its toxemias.

But just what vitality really is and how tremendous it can become; what a higher, superior, absolute health is—has not up to the present date been shown or proven. I will teach in the following lessons a principally different NEW PSYCHOLOGY, based on the correction of medical errors of blood-circulation, blood-composition, blood-building and metabolism. For this purpose it is necessary that you first learn what vitality—what animal life really is.

It is generally admitted that the secret of vitality, the secret of animal life is unknown to science. It will surprise you when shown the truth thru a simple, natural enlightenment, and you must admit at once that it is THE TRUTH. Always remember this fact: "Whatever cannot be seen—conceived at once —thru simple reasoning is humbug, and not science!"

The human engine must first be seen before all other physiological considerations as an air-gas engine, constructed in its entirety—with the exception of the bones—from a *rubber-like, very elastic, spongy material*, called flesh and tissues.

The next fact is that its function is that of a pump-system by air-pressure, and with an inside circulation of liquids, such as the blood and other saps, and that the lungs are the pump and the heart is the valve—and not the opposite—as erroneously taught by medical physiology for the past 400 years!

A further fact—one that has been almost entirely

overlooked—is the automatic, atmospheric outside counter-pressure, which is over 14 pounds to the square inch. Immediately upon, and after each out-breath a vacuum is created in the lung cavity. In other words, the human body animal organism in its entirety, functions automatically by inhaling air-pressure, and expelling chemically changed air and outside atmospheric counter-pressure on the vacuums of the body. That is vitality, animal life in the first instance and importance. *That is "P"*—which keeps you alive, and without air you cannot live five minutes.

But the unseen fact—let us say the secret, is, that it works simply and automatically thru atmospheric counter-pressure, which is only possible because the "engine" consists of elastic, spongy material with a vital strain power—with an ability of vibration, expansion and contraction. Those two facts were the unknown secrets concerning the automatic function of "P" as the phenomena of vitality, and the Chemist Hensel has proven thru chemical physiological formulas, that this special vital elasticity of the tissues is due to a lime sugar combination.

The latin word "spira" means first, air and then spirit: "The breath of God" is in fact first, *good fresh air!* It has been said that breathing is life, and it is true that you develop vitality, health, thru physical and breathing exercises. It is also true that you can remove "O" (obstruction) by higher air-pressure and counter-pressure in this way. It is true that you remove and eliminate obstructions of foreign matter by local and constitutional vibrations, consisting of all kinds of physical treatments. It is true and you eliminate disease matters and obstructions, and therefore relieve every kind of disease thru an artificial speeding of the circulation giving more "air-gas" and vibrating the tissues. You increase "P" (power) artificially for a certain time, but you decrease the vital ability of the function of counter-pressure weakening the rubber-like elasticity of the tissues. In other words, you increase "P" but not "V"—to the contrary—this is done, and can be done only at the expense of "V." You know from experience what happens to a rubber band continually kept stretched or over-exanded. It loses its elasticity.

You relieve diseases, but you slowly lower vitality, particularly of the especially elastic and spongy important organs of lung, liver, kidney, etc. You relieve but do not heal diseases *perfectly*, you lower vitality, just so long as you loosen, remove and eliminate obstructions, exclusively, thru political means (agents) and just so long as you do not stop the supply—the taking in of waste, of obstruction—by wrong mucus-forming, that is—disease building unnatural foods, you lower vitality.

Would any one attempt to clean an engine thru a continually higher speed and shaking. No! You would first flush with a dissolving liquid and then change your fuel supply, should it be a steam engine, the obstructions thru waste being caused through the coal burning only partly.

This involves the problem of dietetics, which culminates in the solution of these questions over its history: WHICH ARE THE BEST FOODS? Meaning, which foods give most energy, endurance, health and increased vitality, or which foods are the basic

cause of diseased conditions and growing old? What
is the essence of life, of vitality, breathing exercise,
activity—a perfect mind or right food?

My formula, the equation shown in the heading,
gives the enlightening answer and solves the problem in its entire mystery. Decrease "O" first by
decreasing quantities of food of all kinds, or even
food entirely (fast), if conditions tell you—second,
stop—or decrease at least by all means obstruction-
causing mucus-forming foods, and increase dissolving, eliminating, obstruction-removing foods and
you *increase* "P," meaning a more unobstructed
function of "P" of air-pressure, of the infinite, in-
exhaustible power source. In other words, the problem of vitality and animal life functioning at all,
consist in unobstructed, perfect circulation by air-
pressure, and in a vital elasticity of the tissues thru
proper food as the necessary counter-pressure for
the function of life.

"P" is infinite, unlimited, and practically the
same everywhere and on everybody continually the
same, *but its activity slows down* in the tempo
(speed) as you accumulate obstructions, as you
over-eat and eat wrong, lowering the automatic
counter-pressure of the tissues.

You may now see that vitality does not depend
immediately, directly and primarily from food or
from a right diet. If you eat too much of the best
ones, especially in a body full of wastes and poisons,
it is impossible for them to enter into your blood-
stream in a clean state and become "efficiency-giv-
ing" vital substances. They are mixed with and
poisoned by mucus and auto-toxemias and actually
lower vitality—they increase "O" instead of "P."

You now see and you may realize very deeply, that it is worthless to figure food values with the intention of increasing "P" or "V" *as long as the body is full of "O."*

This problem is solved by my system, consisting of periodical minor fastings, alternating with cleansing, *not nourishing*, mucus-less and mucus-poor menus. Not as wrongly done with the idea that "V" is directly increased on a sick person thru feeding clean food. Remove "O" thru intelligent, personally prescribed menus. "P" increases automatically after a fast thru its obstructed function. You can now realize how wrong and insufficient it is for people to think that all there is to the "Mucus-less Diet" is knowing the right foods!

Here then, is the cause why so many "Fasting," "Fruit-diet," etc., "cures" fail. THE INEXPERIENCED LAYMAN ALWAYS COMES TO THE DEATH POINT. In other words, he removes "O" too rapidly, too much at once and feels "fine" for a while, the dissolving process goes deeper—"O" increases—he feels terribly weak, falls back on wrong diet, and thus this wrong diet stops the elimination of more obstructions, feels well again—blames the food for his weakness, and sees the wrong food as the food of vital efficiency. He loses his faith and tells you in all sincerity, "I have tried it, but it is wrong." He blames the system, entirely ignorant regarding it, when he alone is to blame. Here is the stumbling block even of other Diet experts and Naturopaths experimenting in dietetics. Lesson 7 will divulge this secret.

Some have had more experiences, but very few think as I do that Vitality, Energy and Strength is not derived from food at all! They believe it is acquired thru sleep, etc. What I have learned and what I know thru years of experimenting, and what I have actually demonstrated, can be found in my book, "Rational Fasting," but briefly stated, it is this:

FIRST—Vitality does not descend primarily and directly from food, but rather from the facts of how far and how much the function of the human engine is obstructed—"braked" by obstructions of mucus and toxemias.

SECOND—Removing "O" by artificially increasing "P" and shaking, vibrating tissues thru physical treatments is done at the expense of "V," Vitality.

THIRD—Vital energy, physical and mental efficiency, endurance, superior health by "P," air and water alone, are tremendous, beyond imagination— as soon as "P" works and can work without "O," without obstruction and friction in a perfectly clean body.

FOURTH—The limit of going without food and before solid food is necessary under such ideal conditions, is yet unknown.

FIFTH—The composition of "P" besides air, oxygen and a certain quantity of water-steam, increases —*but only in a clean body*—by the following other *agents from the infinite:*

ELECTRICITY,

OZONE,

LIGHT (especially sun-light),

ODOR (good smells of fruit and flowers).

Further, it is not impossible that under such clean, natural conditions, nitrogen of the air may be assimilated.

In the following lesson I teach you a NEW but TRUE PHYSIOLOGY of the BODY, which is necessary to know in order to understand why and how the MUCUSLESS DIET HEALING SYSTEM works in its complete perfection, and for this purpose it was first necessary to lift the veil from the secret, FROM THE MYSTERY OF VITALITY.

The New Physiology
LESSON VI

As you now know what Vitality is and how simply animal life functions automatically by air pressure and air counter-pressure, (on fish, etc., it acts exactly the same, by water instead of air), you may realize that medical physiology, the science of animal functions is fundamentally wrong, based on the following errors, which have to be corrected by a New Physiology:

1. The Theory of Blood circulation.

2. Metabolism or change of matter.

3. High protein foods.

4. Blood composition.

5. Blood building.

THE ERROR OF BLOOD CIRCULATION

Medical physiology, pathological physiology, continues to find diseases, the cause of disease—with the microscope, and the germ theory is now in fashion. They will never find the truth and never understand what disease is as long as they have a fundamentally wrong conception of blood circulation.

As I have already explained, the fact has been overlooked, that the lungs are the motoric organs of circulation, and the circulating blood drives the heart—the same as the regulating valve in an engine. That the blood stream drives the heart *and not the opposite*, can be seen thru the two following facts:

(1) As soon as you increase air-pressure by increased breathing you speed the circulation and therefore the number of heart beats.

(2) As soon as you take into the circulation a stimulating poison—alcohol for example—you *increase* the speed of the heart. As soon as you take a nerve and "muscle-band" paralyzing poison, for example: digitalis—you *decrease* the speed of the heart. The Medical Profession have this exact knowledge, but in spite of their knowledge the *wrong conclusion* that a mysterious power acts on the heart muscle driving the blood circulation is arrived at.

Prominent engineers among my patients agreed with my concept after learning this new physiology, saying, that the heart would make a model valve for any kind of an engine.

How can it be logically proven that the heart controls the circulation if thru the circulating blood you can control the heart?

Increased air-pressure thru climbing a hill or running, increases heart action; for the speed of the valve, as in an engine, depends upon the pressure.

Thirty years ago a Swiss expert of physiology, although a layman, demonstrated evidently with animal experiments, that a circulation as taught by physiology and as originated by Prof. Wm. Harvey in London 400 years ago, does not exist at all. Of course no attention was given by medicine to his demonstrations. How can a "science" be erroneous?

METABOLISM

Metabolism, or the "science of change of matter," is the most absurd and the most dangerous doctrine-teaching ever imposed on mankind. It is the father of the wrong cell theory and of that most erroneous, albumen theory, which latter theory will kill and stamp out the entire civilized Western world if its following is not stopped. It will kill you, too, some day, if you fail to accept the truth that a continual albumen replacement is *unnecessary*, and that you cannot gain vitality, efficiency and health by protein as long as your human "engine" has to work *against* obstructions, which are in fact the cause of death of all mankind of the western civilization.

The erroneous idea that the cells of the body are continually used up by the process of life in their essential substance of protein and must be continually replaced by high protein foods, can be and are evidently refuted by my investigations, experiments and observations on some hundred fasters. The facts are as follows, and you will again see that it is just as I teach and as I have experienced. What Medicine calls and sees as metabolism is the elimination of waste by the body as soon as the stomach is empty. Medicine actually believes that you live from your own flesh substance as soon as you are fasting. Even Dr. Kellogg believes that the Vegetarian becomes a meat-eater when he fasts, and Naturopathy has taken over more or less in principle these medical errors. One believes that the human engine cannot run a minute without solid food, protein and fat, and makes the erroneous conclusion that man dies and must die from starvation as soon as all his fat and protein is used up during a fast. I found and have this to state:

Lean people can fast easier and longer than fat ones. The Hindu fakir, consisting of skin and bones, the leanest type in existence, can fast the longest time, and without suffering. Where is there any "using up of the body" in this instance? I further found that the cleaner the body from waste (mucus) the easier and longer one can fast. Therefore a fast has to be prepared by an eliminating and laxative diet. My world record of watched fasting of 49 days could be done under the condition imposed only after using a strict mucusless diet during a long period of time. In other words, I could stand this long fast, and you can stand a fast much easier and much longer the more the body is free from fat—which is partly decomposed, watery flesh—the more the body is free from mucus and poisons, which are eliminated as soon as eating is stopped, entirely or partly. The human body does not expel, burn up or use up a single cell that is in vital condition! The cleaner, the more free from obstructions, from waste, the body is, the easier and the longer you can fast with water and air alone! The limit where *real* starvation sets in is yet unknown! The Catholic church claims tests of holy people who fasted during decades. But the medical error even grows by teaching Metabolism, claiming that you must replace cells (which are not used up as you can plainly see), with high protein food from a cadaver, *partly decomposed meat*, and which has gone thru a most destructive heat process of cooking! The fact is that you accumulate more or less of the wastes in your system in the shape of mucus and its poisons as the slowly growing foundation of your disease and the ultimate cause of your death. Human imagination is evidently not sufficient to conceive the tremendous foolishness of this doctrine and its consequences, unmindful that its teachings are actually said to kill the individual and to finally kill all mankind!

Medicine—and the average man, of course—also believes, that you are growing flesh and increasing health, if you daily increase your weight by "good eating." If the colon of a so-called "healthy" fat man is cleaned of his accumulated feces—even though he has "regular" stools, he at once loses from 5 to 10 pounds of the weight called "health."

Weight of feces, figured by doctors as health! Can you imagine anything more erroneous, more wrong, more foolish, and at the same time more dangerous to your health and life?

That is Medical "science" of Metabolism.

The New Physiology—(Continued)

LESSON VII

3. HIGH PROTEIN FOODS

When the movement for Naturopathy and a meatless diet began in the last century, the men of Medical science were endeavoring to prove by mathematical figures that physical and mental efficiency have to be kept up thru daily replacement of protein with a certain quantity for the average man. In other words—it became fashionable—it became a mania, to suggest and to do exactly the opposite of nature's laws whenever a person felt weak, tired rapidly, became exhausted or sick in any way.

You now know thru Lesson 5 the source of Vitality and Efficiency, and you now know that without food at all, especially protein, the strength of a sick body can be increased.

High protein foods act as stimulation for a certain time, because they decompose at once in the human body into poison. It is a commonly known fact that any kind of animal substances become very poisonous as soon as they enter an oxidation with air, especially at a higher temperature as exists in the human body.

The learned have gone so far as to prove that man belongs biologically in the class of meat-eating animals, while the descendant theory proves that he belongs to the ape family, who are exclusively fruit-eaters. You can see how ridiculous—contradictory —so-called "science" is.

The fundamental fact and truth of why the grown-up man does not need so much protein as the old physiology claims, is shown in the combination of mother's milk which does not contain over 2½ to 3% protein, and nature builds up with that the foundation of a new body.

But the error goes further than that in their endeavor to replace something that is not destroyed, not used up, not "consumed" at all—as you learned in the previous lesson about the medical error of metabolism. The physiology has a principally wrong conception of change of matter, because these "experts," the founders of such a kind of science lacked all knowledge of chemistry at all, and organic chemistry especially. Life is based on change of matter in the meaning of physiological chemical transformation, but never on the absurd idea that you must eat protein to build, to grow protein of muscles and tissue. Most certainly not; for instance, is it necessary that a cow must drink milk to produce milk! A prominent expert of physiological chemistry, Dr. von Bunge, Professor of Physiological Chemistry at the University of Basel, Switzerland, whose books are not endorsing the average standing of medical teaching, says, that life, vitality, is based on transformation of substances (foods) thru which power, heat, electricity becomes free and acts as efficiency in the animal body.

You will learn in the lesson about blood-building that a certain change of matter happens in the human body, and how protein is produced thru transformation from other food substances. This change of matter takes place not by replacement of old cells by new ones, but the mineral substances are the building stones of animal and vegetable life, and the replacement is of much smaller quantities than as now taught.

The reason a "one-sided" meat-eater can live a relatively longer certain time than the vegetarian "starch-eater" is easy to understand after having learned Lesson 5. The first one produces less solid obstructions by smaller quantities of meat-foods than the starch "over-eater," but his later diseases are more dangerous because he accumulates more poisons, pus and uric acid.

If you know the truth about human nourishment —and you are going to learn it later—you will be amused to note how the physiologists grope in darkness—how they made up a standard quantity of necessary albumen for the average man, which standard, by the way, is slowly getting smaller. They, and even advanced "diet experts," estimate without knowing the great unknown: i.e., the waste in the human body. For thousands of previous years man has lived healthier without food value formulas and I doubt very much if a single one of these physiologists ever gave his "chef" a suggestion of food values.

The entire proposition is a farce, masquerading as a so-called science. A few, like Professor Chittenden, found thru experimenting that energy and endurance increased with less food—especially less protein. Professor Hindhede proved that albumen need hardly be considered, and Fletcher outdid them all. He lived on one sandwich a day curing his so-called "incurable" disease and *developed a tremendous endurance.*

After I had overcome all fear as to the fatal consequences that would befall me if I failed to adhere strictly to "scientific protein" necessities, I found, experienced, and demonstrated the hitherto unknown and unbelievable fact that in the clean, mucus-free and poison-free body these foods, poorest in protein—fruits—develop the highest energy and an unbelievable endurance.

If nitrogen, the essential part of protein, is an important factor to keep the human machine running—if vitality depends at all from nitrogen, then it seems to me that under these ideal conditions nitrogen is assimilated from the air.

Food from the Infinite! "P" (power) as a source of nourishment! What tremendous possibilities! I suggest that you read Lesson 5 over again, and you will realize these two facts:

1. The truth about human nourishment is still a "Book with seven seals" to all mankind, all so-called diet experts and scientific experts included.

2. The error of high protein foods as a necessity of health, taught and suggested by medical doctrines to mankind is in its consequences and in its effect just the opposite of what it should be, it is one of the main and general causes of all disease; it is the most tragic phenomena of western degeneration. It produced at the same time the most dangerous, most destructive habit of gluttony; it produced the greatest madness ever imposed on mankind; that is, to endeavor to heal a disease by eating more, and *especially* more high protein foods. It is beyond possibility to express in words what the

error of high protein foods means. Let me remind you that Medicine claims as the father of Medicine that great dietician Hippocrates, who said: "The more you feed a sick person the more you harm him;" also: "Your food shall be your remedies and your remedies your food."

The New Physiology—(Continued)

LESSON VIII
BLOOD COMPOSITION

The logical consequence of the three first errors of the Old Physiology is the problem of composition of human blood—not only as it should be but as a fact of "scientific examination," the error is so great that it borders on insanity.

The problem is this: Are the white corpuscles living cells of vital importance to protect and maintain life, to destroy germs of disease, and to immunize the body against fever, infection, etc., as the standard doctrines of physiology and pathology teach?

Or are they just the opposite—waste, decayed, undigested, unusable food substances, mucus, pathogen, as Dr. Thos. Powell calls them? Indigestible by the human body, unnatural and therefore not assimilated at all? Are they, in fact, the waste from high protein and starchy foods which the average mixed eater of western civilization stuffs in his stomach three times a day? What I call "mucus" as the foundational cause of all diseases?

Pathology proves that itself saying that the white corpuscles are increased in case of disease, and physiology says they increase during digestion in the healthy body, and that they are derived from high protein foods.

This teaching is absolutely correct, and the logical consequence of the error of high protein foods.

Medical "science" sees and must see it as normal conditions of health, and that the non-sick must have these white blood corpuscles in his circulation because everybody has them. There is no man in existence in the western civilization whose body has not been continually stuffed since childhood with cow milk, meat and eggs, potatoes and cereal products. *No man today without mucus!*

In my first published article is the gigantic idea promulgated that the white race is an unnatural, a sick, a pathological one. First, the colored skin pigment is lacking, due to a lack of coloring mineral salts; second, the blood is continually over-filled by white blood corpuscles, mucus, waste with white color—therefore the white appearance of the entire body.

The skin pores of the white man are constipated by white, dry mucus—his entire tissue system is filled-up and filled-out with it. No wonder that he looks white and pale and anaemic. Everybody knows that an extreme case of paleness is a "bad sign." When I appeared with my friend in a public air-bath, after having lived for several months on a mucusless diet with sun baths, we looked like Indians. and people believed that we belonged to another race. This condition was doubtless due to the great amount of red blood corpuscles and the great *lack* of white blood corpuscles. I can notice a trace of pale in my complexion the morning after eating one piece of bread.

This is not the place to bring up all of the arguments against this terrible error about the nature and "function" of the white blood corpuscles believed erroneously by medical "science." Any one desiring a real scientific proof of this, may read Dr. Thos. Powell "Fundamentals and Requirements of Health and Disease," published 1909—a few years after my "mucus theory" was published in Europe, and later translated into English in 1913 as "Rational Fasting and Regeneration Diet," neither of us knowing anything regarding each other's publication. Dr. Powell teaches in principal the same as I so far as the cause of all diseases, the white corpuscles and all these medical errors are concerned. The only difference being that he calls "Pathogen" what I call "Mucus."

In the method of elimination and diet, however, I differ principally and entirely from him; but even in the composition of the red blood corpuscles, the blood plasma at all, the blood serum and the so-called hemoglobein, medical "science" lacks perfection.

The two most important facts for us to know are these:

First—The much greater importance and vital necessity of iron in the human blood.

Second—The presence of sugar-stuff in the blood. That great expert of physiological chemistry and mineral salts theory founder, Hensel, says in his book "Life:" "Iron is chemically veiled in our blood." Doctors could not find it through their lack of knowledge in chemistry. On page 36 of the same book he says: "In our blood albumen is a combination of sugar-stuff and iron oxide, but not to be found or recognized (discovered) in such a way that neither the sugar nor the iron can be found by ordinary chemical tests. The blood albumen must be burned first to make the test perfect."

I presume that the truth and importance is this: The red color of blood is the most characteristic quality of this "quite special sap" and is due to iron-oxide, *rust!* Therefore, it is self-evident how important iron is in the blood. Further—the sugar stuff is of high importance besides its nourishing quality, as it is an essential part in the perfect blood hemoglobin, which if in a perfect state has to become thick, like gelatine, as soon as it comes in contact with the atmospheric air for the purpose of closing a wound. Read in my book "Rational Fasting" my test of a non-bleeding, immediate healing wound, *without* secretion of pus and mucus, *without* pain and inflammation.

One truth regarding the conditions of the human blood found out by doctors is that acidity is a sign of disease. It is no small wonder that this readily happens with the mixed eater, when he fills the stomach daily with meat, starch, sweets, fruits, etc., all at the same time.

Make a personal test if you are not fully convinced. Eat a regular dinner, and one hour after eating get it out of your stomach and you will have a sour fermenting mixture of a terrible odor, reminding you of the garbage pail, and which when fed to hogs causes even these animals to slowly become sick.

Or if you do not care to be so heroic try the following experiment: Next time you sit down to your Sunday dinner have the menu served for an imaginary guest. Empty his portion in a cooking vessel, using the same quantities as you are eating and

drinking yourself. Stir thoroughly. Then cook on
an oven at blood heat for not less than 30 minutes.
Place cover on vessel and leave overnight. When
you remove cover in the morning a distinct surprise
will await you.

The New Physiology—(Continued)

LESSON IX

BLOOD BUILDING

The problem of blood building in the human body involves all problems of health and disease. In other words your health and disease depend almost entirely on your diet; whether you eat right or wrong foods, which foods harm you, thereby building, producing disease, and which foods heal and keep your body in ideal condition, which ones build natural, good blood—and which ones build wrong, bad, acid, diseased blood. These questions and their correct answers are the fundamentals of dietetics and of my "Mucusless Diet Healing System." In this lesson I teach only the principal truth in general. All particulars and details are covered in the entire course.

In fact, my diet of healing in its main and essential part, consists of building a new perfect blood with continual "supply" from natural foods with vital elements thru which the blood stream is enabled to dissolve and eliminate all waste, all mucus, all poisons and all drugs ever taken during a lifetime, wherever and for as long a time as they may have been "stored up" as latent disease in the body.

What the "official" physiology of nourishment teaches for best blood building is doubly wrong.

First, principally as a problem of physiological chemistry. Second, from the truth of nature.

Here again I must quote that great authority of physiological chemistry, Prof. Von Bunge, who personally told me that he does not endorse official, medical teaching. Says Von Bunge: "Life is based on transformation of substances, thru which process power, efficiency, becomes free, just as it takes place in every chemical process of transformation from one chemical entity of atoms and molecules into another one."

The authors that started physiological science lacked, principally, knowledge in chemistry due to a more humanistic education rather than in science of nature. On the other hand, inorganic chemistry was not sufficiently developed at this time.

The misleading idea was again protein. They reasoned as follows: Muscles, tissues, the entire body's essential substance is protein—therefore, this substance must be introduced into the blood in order to build, to grow—in other words, you must eat muscles to build muscles, you must eat protein to build protein, you must eat fat to build fat, and in the case of a nursing mother, she must drink milk to make milk!

As they believed and still believe in metabolism, and the necessity of replacing every day the used-up cells, these principles are followed in the diet of the average mixed eater.

To take inorganic iron, lime, etc., in an endeavor to replace the same substance in the human body is a similar error.

The cow builds flesh, tissues, bones, hair, milk, efficiency, heat, all from grass exclusively. Feeding milk to a cow to increase milk production would be classed as the height of folly, and yet man does this very thing with himself!

Today, every substance of the human body is chemically analyzed and doctors dream of perfecting chemically concentrated food substances in the future making it possible for you to carry your meals in your vest pocket in sufficient quantities to last a couple of days. That will never happen for the human body does not assimilate a single atom of any food substance that is not derived from the vegetable or fruit kingdom.

All manufactured food mixtures, when too concentrated—either of the animal or vegetable kingdom—do not build blood but stimulate only.

Animal foods cannot build good blood; in fact, do not build human blood at all, because of the biological fact that man is by nature a fruit eater. Look at the juice of a ripe blackberry, black cherry or black grapes. Doesn't it almost resemble your blood? Can any reasonable man prove that half decayed "muscle tissues" build better blood?

Just as soon as the animal is killed the flesh is more or less in decomposition. Then they are put thru the destructive process of cooking. No meat-eating animal can live on cooked meat; they must eat it fresh and raw—blood, bones and all.

More complete details about the right and natural foods, will be taught later, and you will learn the truth. I will only mention at this time one important fact, which is essential in my dietetical teaching, and by which I differ from all others, even from other dietetical experts who still believe in concentrated albumen, concentrated mineral salts, etc., being required for good blood building.

Albumen is not the most important substance for our blood, nor is it mineral salts alone which build perfect blood. THE CARDINAL STANDARD SUBSTANCE FOR MAN'S BLOOD IS THE HIGHEST DEVELOPED FORM OF CARBON HYDRATE, CHEMICALLY CALLED SUGAR-STUFF, GRAPE OR FRUIT SUGAR AS CONTAINED MORE OR LESS IN ALL RIPE FRUITS, AND IN THE NEXT LOWER STATE IN VEGETABLES. The newer advanced science teaches that even the small amount of protein that is necessary is developed from grape sugar in the animal and human body. All cereal and vegetable eating animals transform these foods, first into grape sugar, and then as a matter of fact the body in its entirety.

But the essential point of disagreement regarding this particular problem is not in the food, blood-building problem. Whoever does not know disease—latent, acute and chronic, as taught in Lesson 5, will never believe in the truth of human nourishment.

As you now know thru past lessons, just as soon as the blood is improved thru fruits, the average man at once starts the elimination of obstructions —feels better for a while, but when more and more waste is dissolved and with the resultant next shock of obstruction in the circulation, all faith is lost, and he, the doctor, and all, blame the lack of "efficiency" food. He thinks, and every one suggests, that he needs "regular food," which stimulates him for a while and causes him to believe that it must be the meat and eggs that build good blood.

· In other words, the problem of blood building thru right and proper food, the dietetical problem in its entirety will not be solved and the truth will not be accepted nor believed and practiced by those who have not learned what happens, and just what it means to heal by the new and real blood building foods. ·

This is the deeper cause why doctors believe in · and recommend destructive foods, and why the average man keeps them up and increases them continually, for he does not possess the slightest idea of what disease is, and how he daily pollutes his blood.

Critique of All Other Healing Systems and Unbiased, Unprejudiced Reviews

LESSON X

The methods of healing are numberless. Outside of a great domination of superstition in this field, the serious methods can be divided into two principally different classes:

1—MEDICINE
2—DRUGLESS HEALING.

The history of medicine shows that, especially in the past, drugs and other mysterious "inventions" were taken from "quacks." A great number of "medicines," "standard remedies," for example—mercury—were introduced by "quacks." The modern serums, etc., are not better regardless of their being "scientifically" prepared.

As we now know exactly what disease is, we may understand a fact medicine cannot explain, and that is—*WHY* symptoms of disease can be suppressed by drugs and serums to a certain limit. The "results" are known only thru experiences, but medicine does not know *why* these results—"special effects"—happen.

THIS IS THE SECRET: If the body of any sick man endeavors to eliminate poisons manifested by any kind of symptoms and a new and dangerous poison is introduced into the circulation, the elimination thru the symptoms is more or less stopped because the body instinctively sets to work to neutralize these poisons as far as it is possible. The symptoms return just as soon as the life is saved, and the same procedure is repeated until the patient dies—or if intelligent enough—casts medicine aside in time, and seeks to save himself by DRUGLESS HEALING.

The methods of Drugless Healing are also very numerous, and they can be divided into three parts:

1—Physical Treatments.
2—Mental Treatments.
3—Dietetical Treatments.

PHYSICAL TREATMENTS:

In general, all physical treatments have a tendency to loosen local constitutional encumbrances thru various kinds of vibrations and thermal differences. The Kneipp cure, for instance, is in fact an application of artificial colds which stimulates the circulation, and thru that, the elimination.

Exercise (calisthenics), Breathing exercises, Massage, Osteopathy, Mechano-therapy, etc., perform in principle, the same. Chiropractic, however, claims a special "scheme." The subluxation is removed, but Chiropractics, similarly to Drugs, may give immediate successful relief from painful symptoms, but as a matter of fact they return sooner or later, if the adjustments are discontinued, and wrong method of living is persisted in. The cause of subluxation is *an accumulation of foreign matters* between the bones of the spine, and we know that they have their source thru wrong eating, the same as all other symptoms of disease. No doubt the *over-weight of the average man*, in general, is *an-*

other cause of subluxation. Under longer fastings I saw many deformed spines improve wonderfully.

There are various other methods used to shake the tissues and stimulate circulation, i.e., electricity, electric light, sunlight, etc. All of these methods help and relieve, more or less, but *they can never heal perfectly* just as long as they fail to pay sufficient attention to a correct diet; in other words, the elimination of disease or foreign matters will never be complete as long as the intake through wrong foods is not discontinued, and an entirely new blood-building is established through *real, natural* and *clean,* mucusless foods.

MENTAL TREATMENTS:

It cannot be denied that the condition of the mind has an influence on every kind of disease. It is proven that fear, sorrows and worries have a bad influence, not only on the heart and nerves, but on the circulation, digestion, etc. Psycho-therapy, Mental and Divine Healing, Christian Science, have this one great advantage—they save the unfortunate sick from the injuries of drugs! On the other hand, I cannot grant them too much credit, for while they are harmless in a certain sense—they have a tendency, consciously or unconsciously, to keep people in complete darkness as to what disease really is.

We who know exactly, what disease is, cannot agree with a teaching that endeavors to make sick people believe they can be healed by a miracle, or a forced imagination—that they are not sick at all —even though they are actually dying that very minute! It is farcical, not to say pitiful, to pray to the Creator for a miraculous healing—rejecting and disregarding real divine foods—the fruits of the paradise—the "bread of heaven," and instead stuff your stomach three times daily with harmful prepared foods, manufactured by man for commercial purposes, and never destined by the Creator to be man's food at all.

CONFUSION IN DIETETICS

LESSON XI

In this very important lesson it is necessary for me to convince you, once and for all, of the following facts:

FIRST—That in food (in diet) lies 99.99% of the causes of all diseases and imperfect health of any kind.

SECOND—That consequently, all healing, all therapeutics will continue to fail as long as they refuse to place the most important stress on diet.

THIRD—That what I call "mucusless diet" and "mucus forming foods" divides characteristically all human foods into harmless, natural, healing and real nourishing foods—and into harmful, disease-producing ones.

FOURTH—That all other dietetics are mainly wrong because they lay their stress on food values entirely, whether "wrong" or not, instead of the healing, cleaning, eliminating values and their efficiency before the healing process is started, going on, or accomplished at all. (See Lesson 5.)

The dietetical problem, "What shall man eat to be healthy or to heal his disease," is, in fact, the problem of life—as little as it is considered or even known as the most important question. Long ago I coined the following phrase, "Life is a tragedy of nutrition." The confusion and ignorance regarding what to eat is, in fact, so great that it must be necessarily called the "missing link" of the human mind.

That medical science and even so-called "natural" therapeutics see dietetics in general as a secondary question of healing is significant. Even the efficiency of a machine depends upon the quality and amount of its fuel. There is no longer any doubt existing regarding the fact that a plant depends more on the kind of soil rather than climate to produce a high quality of fruit. Farmers understand thoroughly that everything depends on what they feed their livestock. Health and disease of the animal and human body is 99.99% dependent on food. This is tremendously manifested by nature thru the simple fact that every animal refuses food when sick. The animal instinct of responding to every disease or even accident by fasting is nature's demonstration that health and disease depend mainly and entirely from eating or not eating, as well as the kind of foods.

That the average man, and even the reformed doctors, blame everything on earth, excepting food, as the cause of their disease is due to the tragical fact that disease is as yet a mystery in their minds. They don't know how terribly unclean the inside of the body is caused thru the life-long habit of over-eating ten times as much as required—in many cases harmful foods mostly, or even exclusively.

If the average eater, even in so-called "perfect health," fasts 3 or 4 days, his breath and the entire body as well as his discharges are of an offensive odor which signifies, demonstrates and indicates, that his system is filled up with decayed, un-eliminated substances brought in thru no other manner than by eating. This accumulated and continually increasing waste is his latent, unknown "disease," and when nature wants to eliminate by any kind of a "shock," commonly known as disease, he first tries everything to "heal" himself, excepting to fast, to *stop increasing* the cause of the disease—the inside waste.

You have now learned how wrong medicine is, trying to *stop* Nature's healing, eliminating process, called disease, and thereby increasing the inside waste thru drugs and serums. But "natural" thera-peutics of all kinds of elimination will never heal perfectly just so long as you fail to discontinue the supply of inside waste caused by eating and "wrong" eating. You may clean, and continue to clean indefinitely, but never with complete results up to a perfect cleanliness, as long as the intake of wrong or even *too much right foods*, is not stopped.

If it is a fact that food alone is chiefly to blame for all disease—as nature so clearly demonstrates—then it is logical and self-evident that you can heal only by diet; and radically only, if necessary, with the most rational diet; fasting—nature's only "rem-edy" in the animal kingdom.

Therefore, if any kind of diet shall heal it must consist of food, not according to food values as to their nourishing and rebuilding qualities, but ac-cording to qualities of healing, of cleaning, and of elimination.

Here is the cardinal reason why, as well as where, all other dietetics fail. My diet of healing, the "Mucusless Diet," divides, as stated above, all foods, strictly into two kinds: certain ones which heal, and certain ones which produce disease.

It is not sufficient, as the layman imagines, to know which foods are mucusless and which are mucus-forming, but:

1—HOW FAR AND HOW FAST THE CHANGE CAN SUCCESSFULLY BE MADE.

2—HOW THE COMBINATION OF DIFFERENT FOODS HAS TO BE ARRANGED.

3—HOW LONG AND HOW OFTEN FASTING MUST BE INTRODUCED AND COMBINED DURING THE HEALING DIET IF FOUND NECESSARY.

This is the "SYSTEM" of the Mucusless Diet and Fasting, and represents as well what THE PRACTITIONER HAS TO STUDY AND MUST LEARN, and what the layman does not know, and consequently why he must inevitably fail when trying to cure himself with "good foods."

After the foregoing explanation you will at once see in the following critique of the best known dietetics, why they are imperfect, and why the confusion is so great. In later lessons you will also learn of every kind of food, why it is good, and why bad. In case you are still unaware of the foods which are mucusless, and which mucus-forming, they are as follows:

All fruits, raw or cooked; also nuts and green-leaf vegetables are mucus-free.

All other foods of civilization, *without exception*, are mucus and acid-forming, and therefore are harmful.

CONFUSION IN DIETETICS (Part 2)

LESSON XII

The average vegetarian diet omits only meat from the menu, and their mixture of larger quantities of fruits, (good foods), with eggs and milk, cause over-eating—in most cases being *worse* than moderate meat-eating, and a "less mixed" diet.

Three prominent physicians improved the vegetarian diet, but they fail like all other dieticians on the following single point. They believe, more or less, in high protein foods during the diet of healing. In other words—all dieticians without a single exception, outside of myself, think that the body, and especially the sick and weak one, requires "good, nourishing food" to be healed—overlooking the fact that nature alone heals, and does it best by fasting. (Please read Lesson 5 again, so that you may fully comprehend the reason.)

Dr. Lahmann, a German physician, proved in his "The Dietetical Disformation of Blood," that carbonic acid is the cause of all diseases—but he failed to see the deeper cause, the fermentation caused thru mucus-forming foods mixed with fruits. He believed in—and fell a victim to—the protein theory, in spite of his greatly advanced knowledge.

Dr. Haigh, an English physician, with his "Anti-uric acid diet" showed much improvement, but failed in the same manner as Dr. Lahmann.

Dr. Catani, an Italian physician, made up a diet of fruits, green vegetables and meat; eliminating all starch, and healed, more or less, including cases of rheumatism and gout, which Dr. Haigh blamed meat *solely* for these diseases. The secret of Dr. Catani's starchless diet is its laxative effect. It relieves like the laxatives contained in mineral-water springs, but does not heal perfectly. You can see where the point of confusion lies.

Dr. S. Graham, an American physician, whose "Physiology of Nourishment" was fundamental at the time—improved the bread especially; but the improvement consists not in the fact that Graham, Bran and Whole Wheat bread is more valuable than ordinary white bread, but thru its efficiency owing to a less constipating quality than white bread. White flour *makes good paste*, Graham or Whole Wheat flour does *not*. Dr. Graham found an opponent in Dr. Densmore of England, who claimed that over-eating of bran, whole cereals and Graham bread caused inflammation of the intestines. This is, of course, an exaggeration, but Dr. Densmore helped the general improvement of dietetics by advocating more fruits and vegetables.

Dr. Lahmann, the German chemist, Hensel, and some authorities in this country, are the founders of what may be called "the mineral salt" movement. The stress in this dietetic reasoning is placed upon the fact that all acid and mucus forming foods lack the necessary mineral salts. But it proved a fad like the protein fad, thinking health could be regained by overflowing the body with artificially manufactured mineral-salts preparations, and keeping up your old wrong habits at the same time. You improve—relieve to a certain limit, but never heal perfectly.

In a later lesson you will learn how the chemist, Ragnar Berg, improved this "system" to a certain degree. He neutralizes acid-forming foods with mineral-salt-rich ones. At present among the vegetarian health-seekers "Raw food diet" is in fashion. No doubt it represents great progress, but the arguments are partly wrong, and lead to mistaken and fanatic extremes.

They claim all cooking destroys food values, but it should properly be said: "*Wrong* cooking destroys HEALING value qualities (efficiency) of foods, and can even cause them to become acid-forming." The "raw food" experts hint on the same wrong stress, as all others, i. e., The higher food value.

The entire effect or benefit from raw food is the rough fiber of uncooked vegetables which relieves constipation, and acts as an ideal "mucus broom" in the intestines. I do not believe that the human body assimilates "food-value vegetables" such as cauliflower, asparagus, turnips, potatoes, or from uncooked cereals. After a certain beneficial mechanical cleansing of the bowels thru these raw foods the one-sided raw-food eater lacks, in fact, the most important food substance, and that is grape or fruit sugar, unless he eats sufficient fruits.

Significant and instructive is this experiment. Put a lemon in a moderate dry heat a few minutes, and it becomes sweet—like an orange. You develop grape sugar; but let it bake a little too long, or if cooked, it becomes bitter. On the same principle all vegetables when baked improve by developing the more or less starch they contain into grape-sugar. This is true of carrots, beets, turnips, cauliflower, etc.

Raw fruits, and, if desired, raw green-leaf vegetables, form the ideal food of man. That is the mucusless diet. But the mucusless diet as a healing system, uses raw, rough vegetables for their cleansing qualities, baked ones as food, and baked and stewed fruits AS A LESS AGGRESSIVE DISSOLVER of poisons and mucus to MODERATE THE ELIMINATION IN SEVERE CASES. That is one of the most important principles of the system, a point the raw-food fanatic ignores entirely. Eating raw potatoes, raw cereals and unfired pies, is, in my opinion, *absurd* and worse than if they are carefully baked, which means developing the starch into at least partly digestible gluten and grape sugar.

FLETCHERISM

The American, Horace Fletcher, developed a complete dietetical healing system in itself with great success on himself and others. His theory was to eat whatever kind of food you desired, but chew every bite 10 to 15 minutes. You may eat one sandwich a day and get rid of your trouble. The secret is simply this: It is a camouflaged fast; the stomach and intestines have a rest the same as when fasting, and elimination is promoted, and the vital organs recuperate. But when continued longer the bowels constipate from a lack of solid food, and it is said that Fletcher himself died thru severe "trouble" in these organs.

Another camouflaged fast in its effect is the

Salisbury cure. A small piece of beefsteak and a little toast, once a day, nothing else. Relieves, improves, but never heals perfectly.

Under the same classification is the *milk diet*, which puzzles even the most advanced experts of fasting and dietetics by its partial successes in many cases. The secret is this: If you replace three "square" meals a day consisting of at least three courses each, with a few quarts of milk (liquid) the obstructions in the human engine are much less (read Lesson 5), you feel better, and the body partially eliminates, and in many cases, relieves your trouble. But all milk-dieting patients suffer sooner or later from terrible constipation because milk is a first-class, sticky mucus-former.

SCHROTH CURE.

This so-called "dry cure," founded by one of the great Pioneers of Naturopathy, is in its effect also a camouflaged fast. Three days eating nothing other than dry bread, with NOTHING TO DRINK; the fourth day *unlimited drink* of light wine and some food, combined with all-night wet packs. This causes a tremendous elimination, if you can stand the severity of this "horse cure." Schroth had marvelous success and a world-wide reputation, but many who had gone thru this quick help many times, came to my sanitarium and I found they had very weak hearts, and lacked more or less the elastic efficiency of the tissues. Read Lesson 5 again, and you will understand the reason at once. I use the same principles of this cure in an improved form in cases where there was no reaction with a drink fast or by the mucusless diet as follows: Two or three days nothing but dried fruits followed by one day of juicy fruits and starchless vegetables produces a most efficient elimination, but is only advisable for relatively "strong" people.

There are hundreds of other dietetical cures on the "market," and every once in a while one of them becomes fashionable; from the long fast and "fruit fast" up to the so-called "scientifically prepared" mixtures of medical and non-medical dieticians. The average health-seeker thinks that there is some special food or special mixture to be eaten for his particular ailment, and he tries everything— but always in vain, as long as he doesn't know and doesn't understand that there is but one disease— inside dirt, waste and obstructions, and that these obstructions must and can be eliminated only—and systematically only by the opposite of disease-producing, mucus-forming foods, that is, by

"THE MUCUSLESS DIET HEALING SYSTEM,"

a mucusless diet, consisting of fruits and herbs, meaning green-leaf vegetables considered "unfashionable" since the time of Moses, that great Dietitian and Faster. (See Genesis.)

CONFUSION IN DIETETICS (Part 3)

LESSON XIII

After this severe critique of all important dietetics I must admit that I do not deny that all of them have, and have done, considerable good towards the development of the dietetical solution of the food problem and healing of diseases by diet.

Reviewing the entire development during the past 25 years—this fact remains: With the progress of chemistry medical experts arrived at the following conclusion: "We now know exactly all of the elements contained in the human body, and therefore know what must be eaten for upbuilding—for replacement of used-up cells and for producing vitality, efficiency, strength and heat."

You were taught in former lessons why these "conclusions" are wrong, and have produced the "protein" fad and later the "mineral salt" fad, and now the very latest fashion, i.e., the "raw food" fad. Without knowledge of the "great unknown" their conclusions must be wrong. This great "unknown"—unknown to the chemical and medical experts—unknown to the average man and health-seeker—unknown to the layman dietitian—unknown to the general dietetical systems now in vogue—and this "great unknown" is "O" in my formula, "V" equals "P" minus "O"—the waste, the mucus—acids and poisons, the

OBSTRUCTIONS or "O"

in the sick, and also in the average so-called "healthy" human body.

In other words: If human nourishment could ever be figured by mathematical chemical formulas telling exactly what to eat, you will still be fooled by nature—just so long as any ideal food is mixed with, and put into, this waste of mucus and acids already in the human system thru years of wrong living. Nature confuses *you*—so long as you fail to recognize her facts and her truths—but nature herself is not fooled. To the average layman raw food reacts more or less mysteriously—as long as it is mixed with your own mucus—as long as it stirs up mucus and its toxemias in the unclean diseased body and eliminates these poisons. All laymen and experts covering the entire dietetical movement up to the present time, are puzzled, confused, ignorant and still in complete darkness of the fact that in general the average man *first becomes worse*, sometimes developing boils and all kinds of sores— "troubles" up to "indigestion" just as soon as he starts what he believes is a correct and best diet— living on a radical fruit, mucusless or raw-food diet.

"Tell me what to eat," wails the sick, "I want a daily menu for my special disease" (like a drug prescription), and he then considers that as all sufficient. When the elimination sets in he says: "These foods don't agree with me," instead of recognizing that the transition-diet has already started in a moderate way to dissolve and to

eliminate the old waste in the body—with some
disturbance, of course. You must make them realize the necessity of putting up with this temporary
inconvenience, and consider themselves fortunate
indeed to be able to continue with their daily work
instead of undergoing an operation, which would
mean months in a hospital. The foods agree with
them, but they do not agree with the foods.

Now you may understand why the "Mucusless
Diet" is a system in which every change in diet has
certain duties to perform—as a diet of healing to be
applied systematically according to the condition
of the sick.

You will now understand why and in what
manner I differ from all others. The "Mucusless
Diet Healing System" is not a collection of different menus for every disease; it is not "made-up"
combinations of valuable and nourishing foods—it
is not like a medical prescription or a compilation
of standard diets suitable for all diseases, but it is a
system of dietetical changes and dietetical improve-
ments—a system of dietetical elimination of disease
matter, waste, mucus and poisons; a system of
slowly changing and improving the diet as a diet of
healing towards—and up—to the ideal and natural
food of man—FRUITS ONLY—or fruits and green-
leaf vegetables—THE MUCUSLESS DIET.

It is therefore a personally supervised and in
every case different, modified, scientific, systemati-
cal, progressive method of "eating your way to
health," combined if found necessary, with short
or longer fasts.

It is a healing process *thru which every sick
person must go* if he wants to be perfectly healed;
it is an exclusive dietetical "curing and healing,

rebuilding and regenerating process" based on the
use of harmless and natural food for mankind
"coined" and set biologically by the Creator in
"Genesis"—

**"FRUITS AND HERBS," OR
"MUCUSLESS DIET."**

RAGNER BERG'S NUTRITIVE VALUE TABLES

LESSON XIV

You can now understand that the dietetical problem is not solved as the average man imagines thru simply knowing which foods are best and the kind of foods the mucusless diet consists of. You were taught in the previous lesson knowledge unknown to all others—what happens and what must happen in the human body if the sick man eats only the "best foods" or takes a long fast. Later, you will learn how this stirring up and eliminating of mucus by "good foods" and fasting can and must be controlled by yourself, the treating physician or dietetician.

You may now see of what little value and how injurious it may become for the average health-seeker to stuff his stomach daily with terrible mixtures of "good food," "raw food combinations" (in the belief that raw food alone will do it), without any plan or system—without any regard of the disease and his mental or physical condition.

In spite of my antipathy towards "faddists" I will submit a selection of tables prepared by one of the most advanced experts of physiological chemistry —Ragnar Berg, of the special laboratory for food research at Dr. Lahmann's sanitarium of Germany.

Berg's deductions are as follows:

That you must eat as much mineral salt-containing, non-acid producing, alkaline containing foods as necessary to bind, neutralize, compensate the harmful acids, contained in the acid-producing foods which make up the average man's daily menu. In other words—if you want to eat meat, eggs, nuts, milk and starchy foods, you must eat fruits and starchless vegetables to be healthy. It is surprising to note that the majority of foods he calls "acid forming" is what I call "mucus forming," and what he calls "acid binding," that is, non-acid food, is almost exactly what I call "mucusless."

His tables are undoubtedly the best in existence, and their value for us consists in the knowledge of the good and the bad qualities of every food in percentage. He calls it positive and negative properties. You will perhaps be further surprised to note that he endorses and proves by scientific analysis that my classification of harmful foods, mucus-forming and non-mucus forming ones or mucusless diet, is correct and scientifically perfect! He proves scientifically what I had long before found out, that every food which contains and produces mucus after decaying in the system produces at the same time acid. Very remarkable—and important for us to know is what he found concerning fertilizing, and also the result of the average cooking of foods.

Ordinary fertilizing by animal and human excrements, or even by too much minerals—sulphuric acid ammoniac—and superphosphate and by over-irrigating—changes the positive good properties into negative "bad ones," or at least decreases the good qualities. The grower secures the advantage as they look attractive, are of good size and weight, and consequently bring a good market price, costing the consumer more, for food that is really harmful.

This likewise happens thru wrong cooking in too much water—the good qualities go into the water and the present day cook throws these valuable mineral salts away.

As much more fertilizing is done in Europe than in this country, you can readily understand why, especially fertilized rapidly growing vegetables such as asparagus, cabbage, cauliflower, etc., show less value than may be the case with the same variety of vegetables grown here.

In explanation of his tables, Berg states:

"To these various methods of changing healthy foods into poisons belong sulphuring dry fruits, using benzoid of soda or salicylic acid, (both strong poisons), to preserve canned foods from fermentation. The most dangerous one is the method of using the steam of sulphuric acid."

Imagine, if you will, how people are fooled by the showing of big fruit and splendid-looking vegetables—nice bright looking, sulphured fruits.

"The American eats with his eyes," says Dr. Harry Ellington Brook, "preferring snow-white bread, a real starvation food, robbed by refined milling of all mineral salts"—one of the highest negative foods in Berg's tables. Especially, when packed in expensive showy paper boxes, he considers it best, and willingly pays a higher price, little realizing that he is actually "eating his way to death" with these "perfectly combined foods" of modern commerce.

Ragnar Berg's tables of food analysis showing the

positive or good properties, and the negative or bad properties in percentage proves how much acid a food produces (at the same time the amount of mucus), and the percentage of mineral salts of the special kind of alkaline to neutralize acids.

From my standpoint you can see the:

Qualities of a food in percentage to "stir up," dissolve, neutralize and eliminate mucus together with its terrible acid poisonings, stored up in the system since childhood.

These tables by Ragnar Berg were published in Germany 10 years after my "mucus theory" of disease and food qualities had been taught, and Berg unconsciously gave the scientific proof that my "mucus theory" is CORRECT.

The mere fact that some foods given in the list are "acid-binding" does not necessarily mean that I endorse their use. This list is given as a comparison only and should be studied for what it is worth. Undoubtedly by squeezing lemon juice on fish or eating a goodly portion of acid-binding vegetables at the same meal as acid-forming foods are partaken of—the harmful effect is partly lessened.

The higher the "acid-binding" qualities of a food—the more valuable as a mucus-eliminator. Black radish when in season, spinach, dandelion and dill are all excellent internal scourers.

Berg's tables follow:

NAME OF FOOD	PLUS OR ACID-BINDING	MINUS OR ACID-FORMING
FLESH		
Blood of animals	5.49	
Meat (beef)		38.61

Veal		22.95
Mutton		20.30
Pork		12.47
Ham, smoked		6.95
Bacon		9.90
Rabbit		22.36
Chicken		24.32
Ox tongue		10.60

FISH

White Fish		2.75
Shell Fish		19.52
Salmon		8.32
Oysters	10.25	
Herring, salted		17.35
Eggs, whole		11.61
Eggs, white		8.27
Eggs, yolk		51.83

MILK

Milk, human	2.25	
Milk, sheep	3.27	
Milk, goat	.65	
Milk, cow	1.69	
Milk, skim	4.89	
Buttermilk	1.31	
Cream	2.66	
Butter, cow		4.33
Margarine		7.31
Lard		4.33
Swiss cheese		17.49

CEREALS

Refined wheat		8.32
Whole wheat		2.66
Farina		10.00
Barley		10.58
Oats		10.58

Rye		11.31
Unpolished rice		3.18
Polished rice		17.96
Cornmeal		5.37
Pumpernickle Bread	4.28	
Black bread		8.54
White bread		10.99
Graham bread		6.13
Zweibach		10.41
Cakes (white flour)		12.31
Macaroni		5.11

ROOT VEGETABLES

White potatoes	5.90
Sweet potatoes	10.31
Celery roots	11.33
Red beets	11.37
White turnips	10.80
Sugar beets	9.37
Black radish, with skin	39.40
Horse radish, with skin	3.06
Young radish	6.05
Cabbages	4.02
Red cabbage	2.20
Endives	14.51
Lettuce head	14.12
Rhubarb	8.93
Spinach	28.01
Asparagus	1.01
Artichoke	4.31
Chicory	2.33
Tomatoes	13.67
Pumpkins	.28
Watermelon	1.83
Cucumbers	13.50
Red onions	1.09

Kohlrabe root	5.99	
Cauliflowers	3.04	
Brussels sprouts (fertilized)		13.15
Dandelion	17.52	
Dill	18.36	
Leeks	11.00	
Watercress	4.98	
String Beans (fresh)	8.71	
Green Peas (young, fresh)	5.15	
Dried peas		3.41
Beans, dried		9.70
Lentils		17.80

FRUITS

Apples	1.38
Pears	3.26
Plums	5.80
Apricots	4.79
Peaches	5.40
Cherries	2.57
Sour cherries	4.33
Sweet cherries	2.66
Dates, dried	5.50
Figs	27.81
Grapes	7.15
Raisins	15.10
Raspberries	5.19
Oranges	9.61
Lemons	9.90
Pomegranates	4.15
Pineapple	3.59
Banana	4.38
Olives	30.56
Prunes	5.80
Strawberries	1.76
Currants	4.43

Blackberries   7.14
Tangerines   11.77

NUTS
Walnuts   9.22
Cocoanut   4.09
Hazelnuts   2.08
Peanuts   16.39
Almonds   2.19
Chestnuts   9.62

GRAINS, BEANS
Soy beans   26.58
Rye flour   .72
Oat flour   8.08
Oat Flakes   20.71
Sugar Cane   14.57
Rock Candy   18.21

DRINKS
Cocoa   4.79
Chocolate   8.10
Tea leaves   53.50
Coffee   5.60
Chicory roots   7.17
Beer   .28
Porter   2.05
Ale   3.37
Grape juice   5.16
Wine   .59
  "   White California   1.21
  "   Sherry   .51

TRANSITION DIET

LESSON XV

In the preceding lessons you were taught the foods which are best, as well as those which are bad, and which are the worst ones. You know the exact reason why and also what is going on in the system—what happens with good foods as well as with bad ones in the human body. You have learned that even the best foods which have the highest, most vigorous healing properties can become harmful, even dangerous in the beginning, if not carefully used; that they become mixed with the filthy mucus and poisons which they loosen up in the body, and thereby become poisoned, entering the blood stream in this poisoned condition.

Everything is perfectly performed by Nature thru evolutional, progressive changes, developments and accomplishments and not by catastrophies. *Nothing is more incorrect* than the mistaken idea that a decades old chronic disease can be healed *thru a very long fast*, or a radically extended strict fruit diet. "Nature's mills grind slow but sure."

My experience of over twenty years, covering for the most part the extremely severe cases of all kinds of diseases, has proven that a carefully selected and progressively changed TRANSITION DIET is the best and surest way for every patient to start a cure, especially for the average mixed eater. As long as wrong foods (foods of civilization) are partly used, I call it a MUCUS-LEAN DIET. Transition means the slow change from disease-producing foods to disease-healing foods, which latter I call the MUCUSLESS DIET.

The speed of elimination depends upon quantities and qualities of food and can therefore be controlled and regulated according to the condition of the patient. The worst and by far the most unhealthy habit is the HEAVY BREAKFAST. No solid food should be eaten in the early morning at all if you desire to secure the best results. It is permissible to take the drink that you are accustomed to, but nothing else. If you find this difficult to do in the beginning you may drink again later on so that your lunch is taken in the empty stomach. This is so very important that *a number of light diseases can be cured* by the so-called "NO BREAKFAST PLAN" alone. (This subject is more fully covered in Fasting Lessons 17, 18, 19, 20.)

It is best that no more than two meals a day be eaten, even though the quantity you eat is as much as if three or even four meals were eaten. Later, when the stomach is cleaner, a small dish of fresh fruits when in season may be eaten for breakfast if desired. If possible, the first meal, lunch, should be eaten between ten and eleven in the morning, and supper not sooner than five or six in the afternoon. Another very important rule, when eating for health, is SIMPLICITY; in other words do not mix too many kinds of food at one meal. Count the different number of items in the average meal of today and the total will startle you.

NEVER DRINK DURING A MEAL. If accustomed to tea or coffee, *wait a short while after you have eaten* before drinking. Soups should be avoided with meals, as the more liquid taken the more difficult for proper digestion. If a warm drink is desired, for instance, as a breakfast drink during the winter time, make a broth by cooking for a long time different kinds of vegetables, such as spinach, onions, carrots, cabbages, etc., and DRINK THE JUICE ONLY.

Menus for the First Two Weeks

LUNCH: A combination salad, consisting of raw grated carrots or cold slaw or both, half and half, and two or three spoonfuls of a stewed or canned vegetable, such as green peas, string beans or spinach. Add to this one of the following items (whatever is in season): cucumbers, tomatoes, green onions, lettuce or other green leaf vegetables, celery, etc., but only a sufficient quantity for a flavoring.

You may make an oil dressing according to your taste if desired, using lemon juice instead of vinegar—for flavoring purposes only. The rest of the meal should consist of one baked or stewed vegetable such as cauliflower, beets, parsnips, turnips, squash, etc. If you still feel as though you were hungry you may eat a small sized baked potato or one slice of toasted bran or whole wheat bread. Fats of any kind, including the ordinary butter, are unnatural and therefore should not be eaten. However, should you crave fats it is best to use peanut butter or some other nut butter on your bread.

During the winter months canned vegetables may be used when green vegetables are not available. Drink the juice separately in the morning and mix the green or string beans or spinach, etc., with the salad stock as described above of cold slaw or raw carrots. The object of this menu is to supply the "broom" to provide means for mechanically cleansing the digestive tract by quantities of raw, baked and stewed starchless vegetables. This may be called "Ehret's Standard Combination Salad," the "intestinal broom" spoken of so frequently, and so necessary for properly eliminating the stored up poisons now being loosened during the body's house-cleaning.

SUPPER: Mix (half and half) a stewed fruit such as apple sauce, stewed dried apricots, stewed dried peaches, or stewed prunes with cottage cheese or with some very ripe bananas, mashed, sweetened with brown sugar or honey to taste.

The bananas would be for a less "mucused" or less acid stomach.

LUNCH: First a baked apple, apple sauce or other stewed dried fruit. After ten or fifteen minutes a combination salad as suggested in first menu, and bran or whole wheat bread toasted if still hungry. Cow butter should be gradually avoided and replaced by a vegetable or nut butter during the transition. By allowing the cooked vegetables to soak on the salad for 10 or 15 minutes it serves the purpose of a dressing.

SUPPER: A baked or stewed vegetable, as suggested in the first menu, followed with a vegetable salad made of lettuce and cucumber or raw celery or a little cold slaw.

Menus for the Third Two Weeks

LUNCH: During the summer this should be an exclusive fruit meal—one kind only. In winter a sweet dried fruit, for example, prunes, figs, raisins or dates eaten with apples or oranges or the dried fruits can be chewed together with a very few nuts, and then followed by the fresh fruits. If in the beginning this fails to satisfy, wait for ten or fifteen minutes and then eat a few leaves of lettuce or a cold vegetable either cooked or raw, *but just a small quantity.*

SUPPER: A combination salad as suggested in the first menu, followed by a baked vegetable.

Menus for the Fourth Two Weeks

LUNCH: Fruits as in previous menus.

SUPPER: First eat fruits, either baked or stewed, or fresh, followed a little later by a cold cooked vegetable or better still a vegetable salad.

If you find that you are losing weight too rapidly, the elimination should be slowed down by eating bread or potatoes after the vegetables. Should you feel an intense craving, in the beginning, for meat—a great desire returning which you cannot resist, then eat vegetables only on that day, and NO FRUITS.

A Dissolved Mystery

The reason doctors and even Naturopaths in general, as well as the layman, do not believe in a FRUIT diet or MUCUSLESS diet, is simply this: Whoever experiments *without experience* with this diet of healing, whether sick or well, loses his faith immediately, as soon as he has a crisis, becomes what he believes to be "seriously ill," that is to say, a day on which a great amount of dissolved waste, debris, mucus and other poisons are taken back into the circulation, a day of great elimination. This produces at the same time a strong, almost irresistible craving for wrong foods and, strange as it may seem, the patient most strongly craves for the wrong food which was once his favorite. This is explained by the fact that Nature is eliminating thru the circulation the waste of these foods, and it is when they are in the circulation the craving and desire is naturally enough produced.

This then is why it is of extreme importance that every meal of a diet of healing and cleansing *must leave the body* as soon as possible. Being mixed with the loosened and dissolved poisons they cause these "uncomfortable" conditions—a fact that has never before been perfectly understood or explained.

Certain foods prove more laxative under certain conditions. *Therefore, eat the foods that you have personally found to be the most laxative in your own body*. If you do not experience a regular bowel movement before retiring, always help with an enema, a laxative or both. A natural laxative help, which you will undoubtedly find very efficient, is eating a few dried prunes before the other fruits are taken.

A very good aid to elimination which can be used during the transition diet period, until the bowels are cleansed from the old sticky waste, and until such time as the bowels act freely from the new diet is a harmless herb vegetable compound, perfected by myself, and the most efficient intestinal broom and bowel regulator known.

Formula for Ehret's "Intestinal Broom"

Quantities are given in "parts" so that you can prepare any amount that you require.

Note: All "ground" ingredients should be about as coarse as loose tea, the "powdered" ones about as fine as powdered sugar

These are all fairly common herbs and you should be able to purchase them either at your health food store or from an herb shop.

6 parts ground SENNA LEAVES
3 parts ground BUCKTHORN BARK
1 part ground PSYLLIUM SEED HUSKS

1/10th part powdered SASSAFRAS ROOT BARK
1/2 part ground DARK ANISE SEED
1 10th part ground BUCHU LEAVES
1/2 part ground BLONDE PSYLLIUM SEED
1/8th part powdered IRISH MOSS
1/8th part granulated AGAR-AGAR
1/2 part ground DARK FENNEL SEED

Mix the first three ingredients thoroughly. Then combine the remaining seven real well and add this to the mixture. If you have a blender, it makes an ideal mixer for preparing this herbal formula.

The "Intestinal Broom" is easy to use. Usually a small amount, about the quantity that fits on half a teaspoon, or less, swallowed with a glassful of water, is sufficient for adults. It may be increased or decreased according to your own reaction.

Other uses are: sprinkled over salads, or brewed as tea. A half teaspoon to a cup of boiling water, remove from the heat and allow to steep for 10 or 15 minutes. It has a fascinating flavor.

TRANSITION DIET (Part 2)

LESSON XVI

Special Transition Recipes

Being known as a "diet expert" I receive continual requests for a "diet book," or at least a collection of food combinations, mucusless recipes and menus.

Many volumes have already been published by numerous dieticians, which are now on the market, varying in price from $1.00 to $10.00. They call it "scientific diet," but not one of them is in accord with Nature, such as exists in the animal kingdom, and which is SIMPLICITY, with absolutely *no mixtures* at all.

I must again remind you that cattle, for instance, when in the wilderness eat absolutely nothing else than grass during their entire life. No animal when eating combines different foods at the same time or even drinks between mouthfuls of food, with the possible exception of domesticated animals changed into mixed eaters by civilized man.

The ideal and at the same time most natural method of eating for man is one kind of fresh fruit, in season, and you will soon notice after you have been living on the transition diet for awhile, that you will feel more satisfied and in fact are better nourished with one kind of fruit, than with all kinds of scientific mixtures or prepared, made up foods. This condition cannot of course take place until your body is perfectly clean.

During the transition diet I use food combinations and mixtures prepared from cooked, steamed or baked foods for technical reasons, to better perform the healing process intelligently, systematically and under control.

Vegetables and Fruits

My experience has taught me that only *raw* celery, lettuce, carrots and beets combine well with fruits. In general, it is best never to use more than three kinds with the same combination. Always use one kind as the prevailing "stock" or base.

For a bad, acid or "mucused stomach" use menus consisting of more vegetables and very little fruits. For a stomach in better condition, or the average stomach, use more fruits and less vegetables. The following is an example:

1. FOR A BAD STOMACH: Take as stock 2/3 grated or shredded raw carrots, or grated celery or grated beets may be used, altho carrots are best. Add 1/3 of finely sliced very ripe bananas and a few raisins or sliced dried figs. No nuts or cereals. NEVER MIX NUTS WITH WET FRUITS.

2. FOR A BETTER STOMACH: Take as stock 2/3 sliced or grated apples, 1/3 shredded carrots (or celery or beets). To increase the efficiency of this combination in its aggressive, dissolving functions as a mucus and poison eliminator add more raisins, sliced dried figs, honey or a fruit jelly.

Fruit acid dissolves waste and forms gases; fruit

sugar ferments in the waste and stirs it up, also forming gases. Both eliminate and for this reason *it can become harmful* if they work too intensively. It is therefore advisable to use raw vegetables as a "broom" more frequently. For this same reason, use stewed fruits in the beginning, or at least half and half; for example half raw grated apples (with the skin) and half apple sauce, sweetened with honey.

A "Square Meal" Substitute

Before a crisis, during or shortly after, or to satisfy a craving for wrong food especially rich in fat, you may take this once in awhile. While it is too rich it is much less harmful than a square meal and will be found to be very enjoyable:

Take some grated cocoanut, mixed or eaten together with apple sauce, stewed prunes or sweetened apricots.

Very ripe bananas, or if unripened then baked, will be found to satisfy when unusually "hungry."

Other kinds of grated nuts, or nut butter may be served once in a while for this purpose, but are too rich in protein and will produce, if continually used, mucus and uric acid.

Improved "Cooked" Vegetables

Only one kind of cooked vegetable should be used at one meal. It may be eaten either cold or warm, and mixed with green salads and raw vegetables.

If cabbage, carrots, turnips, beets, cauliflower, onions, etc., are slowly stewed in a very little water, or best, if carefully baked, they become sweeter, which proves that the carbon-hydrates are developed into grape sugar, more or less, and the mineral salts are not destroyed and not extracted. This is in fact an improvement and not waste.

In winter canned foods may be used as a substitute for fresh ones. I differ from the raw food "fanatics" because the food value is not important in a diet of healing. It is of more importance that the patient should and shall enjoy his change of diet during the transition until his tastes and conditions have improved.

Special "Mucus-Eliminator" Recipes

1. Raisins and figs or nuts, masticated thoroughly with raw green onions *at the same time*. These must not be eaten separately to secure best results.
2. Grated horse-radish mixed with honey. After mixing allow to stand to take off sharp taste. The honey is only used to make it more palliative. Two-thirds horse-radish and 1/3 honey, or to suit the taste. The ordinary radish, especially the black radish, may also be used the same way, or finely sliced and eaten alone as a salad. For consumptives who cough without spitting, give one spoonful every once in a while. There is a surprising amount of mineral salts in radishes, especially the black radish.

Recipe for a Special Dissolver of Hardened Mucus and Uric Acid

With the following recipe I once healed a woman, who after six years of paralysis, became entirely normal, when both fasting and the mucusless diet failed to effect a recovery. It cannot be taken into a mucus-filled stomach. The recipe follows: Take the juice and pulp of four lemons. Grate and peel of one lemon and mix with the juice. Sweeten with honey, brown sugar or fruit jelly to taste. The object of the sweetening is to make the mixture less sour and bitter.

Dressings

This is really a question of personal taste. A good salad or olive oil with lemon juice to taste is simple and good. A spoonful of peanut butter or nut butter dissolved in water and a little lemon juice added is another simple recipe. Add finely sliced onions (green) if desired. Homemade mayonnaise, using lemon instead of vinegar, is not especially harmful during the transition diet and can be used if you enjoy it. Tomatoes cooked into a sauce, or a good canned tomato soup mixed with the dressing may help you enjoy the "transition diet."

Drinks

Even if the use of table salt is discontinued, you will sometimes be very thirsty during your transition diet, because your mucus, now back in the circulation and the waste of decayed unnatural foods, eaten with salt during your former life is very salty. When in the circulation you will suffer from unnatural thirst. A light lemonade with a little honey or brown sugar will relieve the thirst much better than plain water.

The juice of any of the acid or sub-acid fruits

makes a good drink and the best is sweet apple cider, if not too sweet. Postum, cereal coffee, or even light genuine coffee, if this was your customary drink, can be used during the transition period.

Supplement to Transition Diet Menus and Combinations

The "standard menu" of the day in my Sanitarium, besides special prescriptions for patients under personal treatment, was as follows:

A drink in the morning.

LUNCH: One or two kinds of fruits.

SUPPER: Vegetables, mucuslean or mucusless.

This diet quickly brings the average man, not called sick, into better condition. Slight spells may be manifested in some manner or other, but an "old chronic" or severe disease, caused chiefly thru a drug poisoned body, must be treated by systematically and individually prescribed daily menus, continually changing same, "speeding up and slowing down," according to the patient's changing condition.

The Mucusless Diet Healing System is NOT a propaganda like Vegetarianism or the Raw Food Movement; it is a clinical THERAPY OF EATING that has to be studied and intelligently advised and prescribed personally, the same as is being done by all other methods of drugless healing and therapeutics.

This diet heals every disease if it is possible to be healed at all, because all disease-producing foods are finally eliminated from the diet menus, and the new ones loosen, stir up, remove and eliminate, clean, heal and cure the body.

You build up a new and for the first time in your life a perfect, natural blood composition such as is defined in Lesson 17. This new blood removes and eliminates finally and unfailingly every disease matter even though your doctor failed to locate exactly where it was. See Lessons 3 and 4.

The function of healing, the "operation without the knife," the cleansing, eliminating process begins almost immediately and must of necessity be conducted, controlled and supervised for weeks and even months to secure proper results. The knowledge contained in these lessons is sufficient to enable the student to properly supervise his own individual case.

The menus, combinations, mixtures and recipes are therapeutical adjustments to enforce the self-healing of the body, called disease, and not to suppress or to stop it as is done with drugs.

The average patient expects the right diet to help him at once; therefore the great desire for curative menus and mixtures. Even most of the advanced doctors imagine that a few menus and combinations from one day to the other is all the knowledge necessary.

As yet they don't know the truth that you have learned in the previous lessons, that Physiology and Pathology are fundamentally wrong, that all present day ideas about food and nourishment are entirely wrong and diametrically opposite to the truth. Therefore they do not have the slightest idea what happens and what must happen in the human system, if for the first time in the patient's life the decades old waste and poisons are stirred up and have to be eliminated thru the circulation.

You must realize and perceive that you are starting on an entirely new and perfect revolution, regeneration and rejuvenation of your body, when you change your diet in this way, and it cannot be accomplished within a few days by simply eating some good menus and mixtures.

Mucuslean Recipes

If a little starchy food is eaten after a meal it can be called a MUCUSLEAN DIET. But these starchy foods can be made less harmful by destroying or neutralizing more or less the sticky properties of the pasty starch. The more the potato is baked the better. Toast well done is best.

Raw cereals should be roasted first whenever desired, and will be found to work as a good intestinal broom, altho they contain stimulants. Rice is a great mucus-former because it makes the best paste, but it can be improved by soaking over night in water (you will notice that the water becomes very sticky and slimy and of an awful odor). Pour off the water from the rice and either fry or bake it a little.

A Mucuslean Bread Recipe

Mix a rough bran flour or whole wheat flour with raw grated carrots, half and half, add only as much white flour as necessary to keep the dough, add somewhat grated apples and a handful of grated nuts; also if desired, some raisins. Bake very slowly and well. This is best eaten when two or three days old or well toasted.

Some Improved Recipes of Salad Dressings

Condiments are much less harmful than mucus forming foods. The so-called poisonous table salt is a very good mucus dissolver. The average mixed starch eater could not stand this diet without salt. Of course with the perfect mucusless diet the want and need of salt will be eliminated automatically and with that the unnatural thirst.

MAYONNAISE: Beat thoroughly for at least 5 minutes one egg, to which VERY SLOWLY a few drops at a time one pint of good salad oil (Wesson or Mazola), continue beating while adding oil. Add lemon juice, salt and pepper to taste. If tomato flavor is desired you may add the juices of one tomato.

FRENCH DRESSING: Mix teaspoonful lemon juice, four tablespoons oil, 1/4 teaspoon honey, 1/4 teaspoon of salt, 1/4 teaspoon of paprika. Mix 1 1/4 tablespoons of oil with the dry ingredients, stir well and add the lemon juice. As dressing thickens thru stirring, add the rest of the oil and a little garlic for flavor if you like.

Some Standard Mucusless Cooked Recipes

As I said before you may call the Cold Slaw and Carrot Combination the Standard Transition Salad. Now I will give you the Standard Cooked Mixture.

Serbian Vegetable Goulash

Stew in a very little water or in olive oil or in a vegetable fat coarsely sliced white or red cabbage and some sliced onions with some sliced sweet peppers, when in season, and finish stewing with some sliced tomatoes; a little salt and pepper if desired.

Red or white cabbage with onions baked or broiled in a little fat and tomato sauce as a gravy is an appetizing dish. The same can be done with cauliflower, carrots, brussels sprouts, beets with the leaves, etc.

The idea is to bake dry as possible and to afford occasionally an enjoyable harmless substitute for the chops, roasts, etc., which you have discontinued.

Some Special Suggestions Concerning My "Cook Book"

You will note that all menus and recipes are surprisingly short. If you fall back into the same gluttony-like mixtures, eating foods as described in vegetarian cook books and even in raw food books you will never be perfectly healed. The ideal menu for man is the "mono-diet," consisting of one kind of fruit in season and I must again remind you that no animal in freedom is a "mixed eater" at one meal.

You learned that I use partly cooked food during the transition diet and in the beginning the vegetables prevail. This has for its purpose the slowing down of the elimination, for it is well known that people can stand a stewed or baked fruit whereas they cannot stand the same kind when fresh. Vital food is not the entire object to be gained at first, but rather their property to dissolve and to eliminate. This vital healing efficiency is most perfect in all kinds of fresh fruits and will be found to be too aggressive for the majority of patients. This is undoubtedly the cause of the wrong ideas and reason for the "fruit fast" being in ill repute, and it is the same reason why I use stewed and baked fruits in the beginning to slow down the elimination.

Whenever you feel bad, the cause is that you have too much dissolved mucus and probably old drugs in the circulation; then slow down the elimination by not eating raw fruits, nor even cooked fruits at all and for a few days eat cooked or raw vegetables only. Vegetables work more mechanically and dissolve less.

Later on when the roughest waste is eliminated from your body and it becomes necessary like in all cases of a severe chronic disease to carry the elimination by the new blood deeper and deeper into the tissue system, the diet must be restricted more and more, as the healing process continues.

In the following lessons you will learn how a Fruit Fast must be undertaken, what Scientific Therapeutical Fasting is, and last but not least how the "Mucusless Diet" is properly combined with fasting if found necessary, or the principles and details of the Mucusless Diet Healing System.

The following menus are simply given as examples of how to combine and prepare a meal:

Cottage Cheese and Apple Sauce Mixture—Do not cook apples too long. Use natural sugar sparingly. A few raisins can be added and if desired, lemon rinds or a slice of orange can be cooked with the apples, to flavor. Cottage cheese should be as fresh as possible. Otherwise "smooth" with sour cream or sour milk, stirring thoroughly—or by running thru chopper. Mix together equal parts and serve cold.

A ten-minute intermission affords the family an opportunity of talking over the happenings of the day—always bearing in mind that laughter aids digestion.

Baked Cauliflower—Boil the cauliflower until about half done—then bake in oven until brown. Do not use butter fats when baking but, preferably, Crisco or some suitable vegetable fat. Serve cold, and add dressing to suit.

Salad—Lettuce and sliced tomatoes with peanut butter dressing (made by thinning peanut butter with hot water). Add lemon juice to taste, stirring thoroughly. Then add Wesson Oil slowly, all the while stirring thoroughly.

Bran Bread Toasted

DO NOT DRINK WITH MEAL. Thirty minutes at least should elapse before drinking water after eating.

Raisins and Walnuts (chewed together).
     * * * *
Lettuce, Tomatoes, Cucumbers.
Boiled String Beans.
Baked Potato.
Grapes (if in season).
     * * * *
Lettuce, Watercress.
Radishes.
     * * * *

Swedish Rye Krisp.

Apples, Raisins (always eat fruit first).
Cold Slaw Salad—Slice raw cabbage fine. To soften, add lemon juice and allow it to stand at least one hour before serving. Add onions, chopped celery and boiled cold carrots or cooked green peas. Add mayonnaise or dressing to taste.
*   *   *   *

Baked Sweet Potato (served in jacket).
Whole Wheat Bread (toasted).
DO NOT DRINK WITH MEAL.

Mashed Ripe Bananas, Strawberries (sweeten with honey if desired).
*   *   *   *

Combination Salad consisting of Lettuce, Celery, sliced Cabbage, and cooked String Beans.
*   *   *   *

Whole Wheat Bread toasted.

Cottage Cheese and Apricot Jam (equal parts mixed together and served cold).
*   *   *   *

Lettuce, sliced Tomatoes, ripe Olives.
Baked Potato.

Apple Sauce.
*   *   *   *
Lettuce, grated Carrots, cooked Green Peas.
Whole Wheat Bread toasted.
Baked Apple.
*   *   *   *
Apples and Raisins.

Baked Cauliflower with Peanut Butter Dressing.
Celery.
Toasted Bran or Whole Wheat Bread.

Apple and Celery Salad—Chop apples finely;
chop celery; mix half and half. Add lemon juice to
keep apples from discoloring. Add chopped onions
and parsley to taste. Mayonnaise dressing if desired. (For further particulars see Lesson XVI).
       * * * *
Whole Wheat Fruit Pie.

Baked Apple
Cold Slaw, shredded Carrots, sliced baked Beets,
cooked Spinach.
Oranges.
       * * * *
Lettuce (whole head cut in quarters), sliced
Tomatoes, cooked Baby Lima Beans, green Baby
Onions. Oil dressing or mayonnaise if desired.

Stewed dried fruits (such as mixed Apricots and
Prunes or Peaches and Figs, etc.).
       * * * *
Serbian Goulash (see page 98 for recipe).
Baked Potato.

Stewed Prunes.
       * * * *
Raw Carrots (shredded), cooked String Beans.
Sauerkraut cooked with Apples.
Whole Wheat Bread.
Apple, Celery and Raisin Salad.
       * * * *

Steamed Carrots and Green Peas.

Bran Bread.

Grated Cocoanut and Apple Sauce.

* * * *

Ehret's Standard Combination Salad (grated Carrots, Celery and cooked Green Peas). See recipe, Lesson XV.

Numerous other equally tasty menus can be arranged by simply changing either the cooked vegetable or combination of raw vegetables.

The ideal diet of man is the mono-diet and mixtures are prone to lead to gluttony, so that this should be remembered when arranging the meal.

Note: Prof. Ehret frequently refers to having purposely omitted recipes, in spite of repeated requests, and gave as his reason, "In Nature, such as exists in the animal kingdom, there are absolutely no mixtures at all. The ideal and most natural method of eating is the mono-diet. One kind of fresh fruit, when in season, should constitute a meal, and you will find yourself better nourished. This condition, of course, cannot take place until you have thoroughly cleansed your body of toxemic poisons, mucus, or call it foreign substances."

We feel sure that Prof. Ehret would have approved and granted permission to include a few mucus-lean recipes, particularly of salads, in this edition of his Mucusless Diet Healing System, after being convinced as we have that the public demand requires substitutes from the present day acknowledged method of food preparation, if they are to successfully take up the Ehret method. And so, with this thought in view and with the hopes of converting many more to the Ehret System, we present a few tested recipes; successfully used at Dr. Lust's Yungborn Sanitarium, where the tasty, delicious cooked combinations proved an agreeable surprise to the skeptic.

Salad Recipes

Natural Combination Salad—Large bowl of lettuce cut very fine; 4 handfuls radishes, cut very fine; 4 handfuls tomatoes, chopped; 2 handfuls parsley, cut very fine. Add oil and lemon juice, and mix thoroughly, let stand 15 minutes. Serve with mayonnaise, if desired.

May Salad—Large bowl of chopped cabbage; 1 cup of radishes, cut fine; 1/2 cup sweet green peppers, chopped fine; 1-1/2 cups chopped tomatoes; 1 cup green onions, chopped fine; 1/2 cup parsley, chopped fine; 1 cup cucumbers, chopped —if in season. Mix thoroughly. Add 2 tablespoons lemon juice and 3 tablespoons mayonnaise. Garnish with olives or radishes, for decoration.

Apple and Celery Salad—Two cups cubed apples to which lemon juice has been added to keep from discoloring; 1 cup chopped celery; 1/4 cup fine chopped parsley; 1 handful seedless raisins; 2 tablespoons mayonnaise, mixed thoroughly. Serve on crisp lettuce leaves.

Cabbage Salad (delicious)—Two cups shredded cabbage; 1 cup finely chopped green peppers; 1/2 cup chopped almonds; 1 tart apple, cut in strips about 1 inch long. Salt to taste. Add 2 tablespoons lemon; soak 10 minutes. Add 2 tablespoons mayonnaise dressing. Mix thoroughly. Serve on crisp lettuce leaves. Decorate with chopped pimiento.

Carrot and Raisin Salad—Two cups coarsely shredded carrots. Soak 1/2 cup seedless raisins about 2 hours; 1/2 cup finely chopped celery. Mix thoroughly. Add 2 tablespoons mayonnaise.

Stuffed Prune Salad—Fill centers of cooked prunes with cottage cheese. Place 1 blanched almond in center of cottage cheese. Serve on lettuce leaves with mayonnaise.

Cooked Combination Salad—One cup diced cooked carrots; 1 cup cooked peas; 1 cup chopped cooked string beans; 1/2 cup finely chopped raw celery. Mix thoroughly; add mayonnaise. Serve on crisp lettuce leaves.

Serbian Slaw—One cup coarsely chopped celery; 1 cup finely sliced cabbage; 1/4 cup finely chopped onions; 1/4 cup minced olives; tablespoon chopped pimiento. Add oil and lemon juice.

Fruit Salad (served in Apple Shells)—Select good looking apples. Cut off piece of top and remove meat of apple. Chop together the apple hearts, pineapple and grapefruit, and cherries, in equal parts. Add lemon juice. Sweeten with honey and place in the shells of apples. Sprinkle with grated cocoanut.

Mexican Cold Slaw—Two cups of finely sliced red

cabbage; 1/2 cup chopped celery; 1 cup red kidney beans; 1/4 cup chopped onions; 1/4 cup chopped peppers. Add olive oil and lemon juice.

Carrot and Apple Salad—One cup chopped carrots; 1 cup cubed apples, soaked in lemon juice; 1/2 cup chopped celery; finely chopped onions to flavor; 1/2 cup finely sliced dates. Add olive oil and lemon juice. Soak for 15 minutes. Serve on crisp lettuce leaves.

Summer Salad—One cup chopped water cress; 1/2 cup chopped tomatoes; 1/2 cup diced cucumbers; 1/2 cup diced celery. Add olive oil and lemon juice. Mix thoroughly and serve on crisp lettuce leaves.

Russian Salad—Two ripe tomatoes; 4 medium size carrots, diced; 1/2 finely chopped onion; 2 sprigs chopped water cress; 2 stalks celery, cut in 1-inch lengths and split. Mix with mayonnaise. Serve on bed of lettuce. Garnish with sliced tomatoes.

Asparagus Salad—Cook asparagus and cut into 3-inch lengths. Make bed of finely sliced lettuce. Put asparagus on lettuce. Add mayonnaise if desired.

Cauliflower and Pea Salad—Soak cauliflower and break into small pieces. To 2 cups cauliflower, add 1 cup cooked peas and 1 cup chopped parsley. Add mayonnaise and serve on lettuce leaves.

Asparagus and Cauliflower Salad—Boil asparagus

and cut tips in 3-inch lengths. Boil cauliflower and break in small pieces. Mix together in equal portions. Add mayonnaise. Serve on lettuce leaves.

Brazilian Salad—One and one-half cups ripe strawberries; 1-1/2 cups cubed pineapple, fresh; 12 blanched thinly sliced Braxil nuts; marinated in 4 tablespoons of lemon juice. Arrange lettuce on plates in rose shape. Fill crown with above mixture. Cover with spoonful of mayonnaise. Decorate with strawberries.

Date and Celery Salad—Chop dates and celery—equal parts. Serve with mayonnaise, on lettuce.

Waldorf Salad—One and one-half cups diced apples; 1/2 cup lemon juice; 1-1/4 cups diced celery. Mix apples, celery and lemon juice well together. Use crisp, tart apples. Drain off lemon juice. Add mayonnaise dressing. Serve on crisp lettuce. Decorate with grated walnuts.

Mock Chicken Salad—Two cups finely sliced cabbage; 1 cup celery; 2 tablespoons finely chopped onion; 1/2 cup green peppers, finely chopped; 1 cup cubed nut loaf, cold. Add 2 tablespoons mayonnaise. Mix thoroughly. Serve on crisp lettuce leaves. Decorate with olives.

Grated Carrot and Spinach Salad—One cup grated carrots; 1 cup chopped spinach; 1 cup cold slaw. Add lemon juice to spinach and cold slaw, and soak 10 minutes. Prepare salad plates with leaves of crisp lettuce—bottom layer cold slaw, second layer chopped spinach. Top layer grated carrots. One spoonful mayonnaise, and ripe olive in center for decoration.

Elimination Salad—Two cups chopped spinach; 2 cups cold slaw; 1 cup fresh green peas; 1 cup chopped celery. Mix thoroughly. Add lemon juice and oil. Serve as desired.

Water Cress Salad—Make bed of lettuce. Chop water cress. 2 tomatoes, sliced.

Mixed Salad—Chop lettuce leaves (1 large bowl); 2 cups chopped tomatoes; 1 cup chopped celery; 1 cup chopped onions; 1/2 cup chopped parsley. Mix thoroughly. Add lemon juice and oil.

Onion Salad—Two cups finely sliced cabbage; 1 cup sliced red onions; 1 cup chopped tomatoes; 1/2 cup coarsely chopped parsley. Add 2 table-spoons mayonnaise and mix thoroughly. Serve on crisp lettuce leaves. Decorate with radishes.

Cooked Vegetable Recipes

Mock Ham Loaf—One pound nut meat substitute; 1/4 lb. protose; 4 teaspooons Savita or Vegex; 1/2 teaspoon salt; 3 tablespoons margarine; 1 table-spoon onion juice; 1/4 oz. Vegex gelatine; 1 cup boiling water. Mix 1/2 lb. of the nutmeat with 2 tablespoons margarine. Set aside to use later. To prepare gelatine: Soak for 30 minutes in warm water. Remove from water and put to cook in boiling water for 8 minutes boiling. Strain. Cook in the boiling water. Mince the protose and mix with all other ingredients. Set on ice. When cold cover with nutmeat and butter. Cut in slices. Garnish with a spray of parsley.

Stuffed Onions—Select good sized onions. Remove slice from top of each onion. Parboil onions until almost tender. Strain and remove centers, making six cups. Chop onion that was scooped out. Combine with soft crumbs and protose, or chopped pepper and tomato pulp. Add seasoning to taste. Refill onion cups. Place in pan and cover with onion crumbs. Add 1/2 cup milk. Bake until tender.

Protose Cutlets—One pound savory loaf; 1 cup bran flakes; 2 cups milk; 2 eggs; 1 teaspoon salt. Cut can of protose in halves and each half into 12 slices. Sprinkle bottom of dripping pan with 1/2 of bran flakes. Beat eggs until whites and yolks are well blended; add milk and salt. Pour over savory loaf. Bake in very slow oven until set.

Spinach Loaf—Wash spinach thoroughly. Cook in its own juice until tender. Drain and chop. Chill and add onion finely chopped, and the celery, finely cut. Moisten with French dressing. Mold and bake in pan. Garnish with hard boiled eggs if desired. Serve hot or cold.

Protose Hash—One and one-half cups protose; 2 cups potatoes, cold, boiled or baked; 4 tablespoons oil; 2 onions, chopped; salt; 2 tablespoons flour. Brown wholewheat flour and onions in oil; add 2 cups hot water; cook until done. Add remainder of ingredients and bake until brown.

Protose Stew—One tablespoonful butter; 1 tablespoonful parsley, minced; 4 cups strained tomatoes; 4 onions; 2 tablespoons flour; 1 lb. protose. Put butter in saucepan. Add sliced onion and parsley and cook 10 minutes. Stir in flour and mix thoroughly. Add tomatoes. Stir well to free from lumps. Cover and cook 20 to 30 minutes. Slice protose into small pieces and simmer in sauce 10 minutes. Salt and serve.

Vegetable Oysters (Stew)—Oyster plant, cut in 1/4-inch slices, 1 quart; 2 cups milk; 1 tablespoon butter; salt to taste. Wash and scrape oyster plant, slice and put in cold water to prevent discoloration. Cook in sufficient water to cover. When tender, drain, add milk and butter. Let simmer a few minutes and serve.

New England Boiled Dinner—Four and one-half cups potatoes; 1 cup turnips; 2 cups onions; 1-3/4 cups carrots; 2-1/2 cups cabbage. Cut potatoes, carrots and turnips in 3/4-inch cubes. Slice onions. Cut cabbage into pieces about 1-1/2 inches square. Boil potatoes and onions together. Cabbage may be either cooked separately or added to carrots and turnips when they are partially cooked. When all are done, mix together and serve with slices of protose or other nut food that has been braised in a tomato, or brown sauce.

Baked Artichokes—Boil until done. Remove from water. Spread open a few of outside leaves and add garlic cloves. Place in pan. Pour over olive oil and bake in oven about 25 minutes.

Baked Egg Plant—One quart diced egg plant; 1 cup milk; 1 egg; 2 teaspoons butter; 2 cups bread crumbs, toasted; 1/2 teaspoon salt; Nucoa. Peel egg plant, cut into 3/4-inch cubes. Soak in cold water to which 1 teaspoon salt to 1 quart water has been added. Soak 1/2 hour or more. Drain. Cook in boiling salted water. When tender, drain. Add beaten egg slowly, then salt and milk. Pour over egg plant. Melt in nucoa and stir in crumbs. Add buttered crumbs and bake on oiled pan in moderate oven until set.

Egg Plant Hash—Cut in half lengthwise. Place in oven until baked to a mushy pulp. Remove the peel. Mash. Add fried onion. Season with butter, salt and pepper.

Baked Beet Tops—Boil beet tops and spinach separately, half of each. Drain and chop. Braise onions. Add chopped celery. Mix all together. Put in pan. Cover with bread crumbs and bake.

Vegetable Chicken a la King—Two stalks sliced celery; 2 cups chopped bell peppers; 1/4 cup pimiento; 1/2 cup green peas; 1/2 cup carrots, cubed. Add sliced onion. Make cream wholewheat flour gravy. Serve on wholewheat toast or patties.

Mock Chicken Croquettes—Make base of braised onions, bell peppers and celery. Add mashed baked potatoes, carrots, peas—or other cooked vegetables if preferred. Toasted bread crumbs. Mold and bake in Crisco until golden brown.

Vegetable Chop Suey—Braise coarsely chopped onions. Put in pot to bake. Add chopped celery, bean sprouts, chopped bell peppers, water chestnuts, dried mushrooms (soak mushrooms at least three hours before using), tomatoes to flavor. Add diced protose. Bake as dry as possible.

Mock Country Sausage—Boiled brown rice; bread crumbs, toasted; celery; chopped walnuts; peanut butter; sliced onions braised in Vegex. Flavor with garlic and sage. Salt to flavor. Mold in round balls. Bread and dip in hot Crisco until golden brown.

Vegetable Hamburger—Braise onions with bell peppers. Add garlic to taste. Cook together. Add toasted bread crumbs, celery, walnuts and hominy. Mold and bake in oiled pan. Serve with onions.

Stuffed Bell Peppers—Four large peppers; 1-1/2 tablespoons margarine; 1-1/2 tablespoons whole-wheat flour; 1 cup milk; 1/2 cup chopped nut meats; 1 cup bread crumbs; 1/2 cup diced celery; 4 teaspoons grated onion. Remove seeds from peppers and parboil 10 minutes. Drain. Make sauce of margarine, flour and milk. Add chopped nut meats, celery and grated onion. Season to taste with salt and pepper. Fill cooked drained peppers with mixture. Spread additional crumbs on top of peppers. Bake in Crisco or margarine.

Baked Tomatoes—Cut tops from tomatoes and scoop out pulp. Season pulp with grated onions and parsley. Replace into shells of tomatoes, put tops back on, cover and bake for 25 minutes, basting with good salad oil. Arrange on bed of water cress or lettuce surrounded by sliced cooked beets. Use dressing desired.

Carrot Nut Loaf—Two cups coarsely chopped carrots; 1/2 cup Zo crumbs; 1 cup chopped celery; 3/4 cup chopped walnuts; 1 cup mashed tomatoes; 1/2 cup braised sliced onions. Mix together, add 2 tablespoons margarine. Place in loaf pan and bake 1/2 hour.

Vegetable Sausage and Sauerkraut—One cup sliced onions; 2 cups natural brown rice; 1/4 cup finely chopped peanuts; 1/2 cup Zo crumbs. Braise onions in margarine. Soak rice over night, or at least 6 hours, and after pouring off water, add fresh water and boil until soft. Mix rice, Zo, peanuts and onions. Mold in shape of sausages, dip in egg and roll in fine cracker crumbs. Dip in hot Crisco until golden brown. Warm sauerkraut and serve.

Zuccini-Italienne—Slice in about 1/2-inch thickness 2 good sized zuccini; 1 good sized tomato; 1/2 red onion, sliced; and 1 small clove of garlic, if desired. Cook zuccini and onions for about 30 minutes, add tomatoes and cook additional 10 minutes.

New Potatoes and String Beans—Steam potatoes and peel. Cook string beans with as little water as possible. Place both on baking pan and add chopped parsley. Pour over Italian Olive Oil and warm in oven for 15 minutes. Serve.

Corn Saute—Two cups shoepeg corn; 1/4 cup chopped bell peppers (braised); 1/4 cup chopped onions; 1/8 cup chopped pimientos. Mix ingredients and bake 15 minutes in a slow oven.

Vegetarian Corn Beef—One cup of cubed carrots; 1 cup of cabbage, coarsely chopped; 1 cup nut meat Savory loaf; 1/2 cup potatoes; 1/2 cup celery chopped. Steam vegetables. Fill baking pan 1/2 full with brown gravy, add ingredients, brush lightly with margarine, and bake 10 minutes at 400 degrees Fahrenheit.

Italian Meat Balls—Soak spaghetti (wholewheat) and cook until tender, about 2 cups; 2 cups of nut meat loaf; 1/2 cup onions; 1/2 cup chopped celery; 1/8 cup hot peppers, or to flavor. Mix ingredients, after adding Spanish sauce. Form in balls, bake in pan and serve with Spanish sauce.

Mock Halibut Cutlets with Tartar Sauce—Two cups lima beans; 1/2 cup sliced onions; 1/2 cup bell peppers; 1/2 cup farina. Boil lima beans until soft, braise onions and bell peppers together with Vegex flavoring. Mix ingredients, dip in bread crumbs and bake after molding in any form desired. Serve with tartar sauce made without vinegar or pickles, and sprigs of parsley.

Nut Loaf—One cup hot cooked brown rice; 1 cup chopped walnut or pecan meats; 1 cup wholewheat cracker crumbs; 1 egg; 1 cup milk; 1 tablespoon melted margarine. Mix rice, chopped nuts, crumbs and then add beaten egg, milk and salt to taste.

Turn mixture into greased loaf pan, pour over margarine, cover and bake 1 hour moderate oven. Serve with tomato sauce.

Nut Lisbon Steak—Two cups boiled brown rice, cold; 1 cup braised sliced onions; 1/4 cup chopped walnuts or pinenuts. Mix thoroughly. Mold and dip in or wipe with egg, dip in fine wholewheat cracker crumbs. Dip in boiling Crisco until golden brown.

FASTING (Part 1)

LESSON XVII

It is significant for our time of degeneration that fasting, by which I mean living without solid and liquid food, is still a problem as a healing factor for the average man, as well as for the orthodox medical doctor. Even Naturopathy required a few decades in its development to take up Nature's only, universal and omnipotent "remedy" of healing. It is further significant that fasting is still considered as a "special" kind of cure, and due to some truly "marvelous" results here and there, it has quite recently become a world-wide fad. Some expert Nature-cure advocators plan out general "prescriptions" of fasting, and how to break a fast regardless of your condition or the cause from which you are a sufferer.

On the other hand, fasting is so feared and misrepresented that the average man actually considers you a fool if you miss a few meals when sick, thinking you will starve to death, when in reality you are being cured. He fails to understand the difference between fasting and starvation. The medical doctor in general endorses and, in fact, teaches such foolish beliefs regarding Nature's only foundational law of all healing and "curing."

117

Whatever has been designed and formulated to eliminate the disease matters and designed as "natural treatments" without having at least some restriction or change in diet, or fasting, is a fundamental disregard of the truth concerning the cause of disease.

Have you ever thought what the lack of appetite means when sick? And that animals have no doctors, and no drug stores, and no sanitariums, and no machinery to heal them? Nature demonstrates and teaches by that example that there is only one disease and that one is caused thru eating and, therefore, every disease whatsoever it may be named by man, is and can be healed by one "remedy" only—by doing the direct opposite of the cause—by the compensation of the wrong—*i.e.*, reducing the quantity of food or fasting. The reason so many, and especially long fasting, cures have failed and continue to fail is due to the ignorance which still exists regarding what is going on in the body during a fast, an ignorance still existing even in the minds of Naturopaths and fasting experts up to the present date.

I dare say there may not be another man in history who has studied, investigated, tested and experimented on fasting as much as I did. There is no other expert at present, as far as I know, who conducted so many fasting cures on the most severe cases, as I did. I opened the first special sanitarium in the world for fasting, combined with the Mucusless Diet, and fasting is an essential part of the Mucusless Diet Healing System. I have likewise made four public scientific tests of fasting of 21, 24 and 32 days, respectively, as a demonstration. The latter test is the *world's record* of a fast conducted under a strict *scientific supervision of government officials.*

You may therefore believe me when I teach something new and instructive about what actually happens in the body during a fast. You learned in Lesson 5 that the body must first be considered as a machine, a mechanism made of rubber-like material which has been over-expanded during its entire life thru overeating. Therefore, the functioning of the organism is continually obstructed by an unnatural over-pressure of the blood and on the tissues. As soon as you stop eating, this over-pressure is rapidly relieved, the avenues of the circulation contract, the blood becomes more concentrated and the superfluous water is eliminated. This goes on for the first few days and you may even feel fine, but then the obstructions of the circulation become greater because the diameter of the avenues becomes smaller and the blood must circulate thru many parts of the body, especially in the tissues, at and around the symptom, against sticky mucus pressed-out and dissolved from the inside walls; in other words, the blood stream must overcome, dissolve and carry with itself mucus and poisons for elimination thru the kidneys.

When you fast you eliminate first and at once the primary obstructions of wrong and too much eating. This results in your feeling relatively good, or possibly even better than when eating, but, as previously explained, you bring new, secondary obstructions from your own waste in the circulation and you feel miserable. You and everyone else blames the lack of food. The next day you can notice with certainty mucus in the urine and when the quantity of waste, taken in the circulation, is eliminated, you will undoubtedly feel fine, even stronger than ever before. So it is a well known fact that a faster can feel better and is actually stronger on the twentieth day than on the fifth or sixth day, certainly a *tremendous* proof that *vitality does not depend primarily on food*, but rather from an unobstructed circulation. (See Lesson 5.) The smaller the amount of "O" (obstruction) the greater "P" (air pressure) and therefore "V" (vitality).

Thru the above enlightening explanation you see that fasting is: first, a negative proposition to relieve the body; second, that it is a mechanical process of elimination by from direct obstructions of solid, most unnatural foods; contracting tissues pressing out mucus, causing friction and obstruction in the circulation.

The following are examples of vitality from "P," Power, air pressure alone:

One of my first fasters, a relatively healthy vegetarian, walked 45 miles in the mountains on his 24th fast day.

A friend fifteen years younger and myself walked 56 HOURS CONTINUALLY after a ten-day fast.

A German physician, a specialist in fasting-cures, published a pamphlet entitled, "Fasting, the Increase of Vitality." He learned the same fact that I did, but he does not know why and how, and vitality therefore remained mysterious for him.

If you drink only water during a fast, the human mechanism cleanses itself, the same as though you would press out a dirty watery sponge, but the dirt in this instance is sticky mucus, and in many cases pus and drugs, which must pass thru the circulation until it is so thoroughly dissolved that it can pass thru the fine structure of the "physiological sieve" called kidneys.

FASTING (Part 2)

LESSON XVIII

As long as the waste is in the circulation you feel miserable during a fast; as soon as it is thru the kidneys you feel fine. Two or three days later and the same process repeats itself. It must now be clear to you why conditions change so often during a fast; it must now be clear to you why it is possible for you to feel unusually better and stronger on the twentieth fast day than on the fifth, for instance.

But this entire cleansing work, thru continued contracting of the tissues (becoming lean) must be done by, and with the original old blood composition of the patient, and consequently a long fast, especially a too long fast, may become in fact a crime if the sick organism is too greatly clogged up by waste. Fasters who died from too long a fast did not die from lack of food, but actually suffocated in and with their own waste. I made this statement years ago. More clearly expressed: The immediate cause of death is not a poverty of the blood in vital substances, but from too much obstruction. "O" (obstruction) becomes as great as or even greater than "P" (air pressure) and the body mechanism is at its "death point."

I gave all of my fasters lemonade with a trace of

honey or brown sugar for loosening and thinning the mucus in the circulation. Lemon juice and fruit acids of all kinds neutralize the stickiness of mucus and pus (acid paste cannot be used for sticking purposes).

If a patient has ever taken drugs over his entire life period—which are stored up in the body like the waste from food, his condition might easily become serious or even dangerous when these poisons enter the circulation, when he takes his first fast. Palpitation of the heart, head aches, nervousness may set in, and especially insomnia. *I saw patients eliminate drugs they had taken as long as forty years before.* Symptoms such as described above are blamed on the "fast" by everybody, and especially doctors.

How Long Should One Fast?

Nature answers this question in the animal kingdom with a certain cruelty, "fast until you are either healed or dead!" In my estimation 50 to 60% of the so-called "healthy" men of today and 80 to 90% of the seriously chronic sick would die from their latent diseases thru a long fast.

How long one should fast cannot be definitely stated at all, in advance, even in cases where the condition of the patient is known. When and how to break the fast is determined by noting carefully *how conditions change during the fast*—you now understand that the fast should be broken *as soon as you notice that the obstructions are becoming too great* in the circulation, and the blood needs new vital substances to resist and neutralize the poisons.

Change your ideas regarding the claim "the longer you fast the better the cure." You may now readily understand why. Man is the sickest animal on earth; no other animal has violated the laws of eating as much as man; no other animal eats as wrongly as man.

Here is the point where human intelligence can correctively assist in the self-healing process by the following adjustments which embrace the Mucusless Diet Healing System:

First. Prepare for an easier fast by a gradually changing diet towards a mucusless diet, and by laxatives and enemas.

Second. Change shorter fasts periodically with some eating days of cleansing mucus-poor and mucusless diet.

Third. Be particularly careful if the patient used much drugs; especially if a mercury or saltpetre, oxide of silver (taken for venereal diseases) have been used, in which case a long, slowly changing, preparative diet is advisable.

An "expert's" suggestion to fast until the tongue is clean caused many troubles with "fanatical" fasters, and I personally know of one death. You may be surprised when I tell you that I had to cure patients from the ill-effects of too long a fast. The reason will be clear later.

In spite of the above, every cure, and especially every cure of diet should start with a two or three-day fast. Every patient can do this without any harm, regardless of how seriously sick he may be. First a light laxative and then *an enema daily*, makes it easier as well as harmless.

How to Break a Fast

The right food after a fast is as important and decisive for proper results as the fast itself. At the same time, it depends entirely upon the conditions of the patient, and very much upon the length of the fast. You may learn from the results of the two extreme cases, both of which ended fatally (not from the fast, but from the first wrong meal), just why this KNOWLEDGE *is so important.*

A one-sided meat eater, suffering from diabetes, broke his fast which lasted about a week by eating dates and died from the effects. A man of over 60 years of age fasted twenty-eight days (too long); his first meal of vegetarian foods consisting mainly of boiled potatoes. A necessary operation showed that the potatoes were kept in the contracted intestines by thick sticky mucus so strong that a piece had to be cut off, and the patient died shortly after the operation.

In the first case the terrible poisons loosened in the stomach of this one-sided meat eater during his fast when mixed with the concentrated fruit sugar of the dates caused at once so great a fermentation with carbonic acid gases and other poisons that the patient could not stand the shock. The correct advice would be: First a laxative, later raw and cooked starchless vegetables, a piece of rough bran bread toast. Sauerkraut is to be recommended in such cases. No fruits should be eaten for a long time after fast has been broken. The patient should have been prepared for the fast by a longer transition diet.

In the second case the patient fasted entirely too long for a man of his age without proper preparation. Hot compresses on the abdomen, high enemas might have helped the elimination, together with a strong eliminative laxative and then starchless, mostly raw, vegetables; no fruits for a considerable time.

Thru these two very instructive examples you may see how individually different the advice must be, and how wrong it is to make up general suggestions concerning how to break a fast.

FASTING (Part 3)

LESSON XIX

Important Rules to be Carefully Studied and Memorized

What can be said in general, and what I teach is new and different from the average fasting experts, and is as follows:

1. The first meal and the menus for a few days after a fast must be of a laxative effect, and not of nourishing value as mostly all others think.

2. The sooner the first meal passes thru the body the more efficiently it carries out the loosened mucus and poisons of the intestines and the stomach.

3. If no good stool is experienced after two or three hours, help with laxatives and enemas. Whenever I fasted I always experienced a good bowel movement at least one hour after eating, and at once felt fine. After breaking a long fast I spent more time on the toilet than in bed the following night—and that was as it should be.

While sojourning in Italy many years ago, I drank about three quarts of fresh grape juice after a fast. At once I experienced a watery diarrhea set in foaming mucus. Almost immediately after I experienced a feeling of such unusual strength that I easily performed the knee-bending and arm-stretching exercise 352 times. This removal thoroughly of obstructions, taking place after a fast of a few days, increased "P"—vitality at once! You will have to experience a similar sensation to believe me, and then you will agree with my formula, "V" = "P" – "O," and you will realize the absurdity of making up scientific nourishing menus for health and efficiency.

4. The longer the fast the more efficiently the bowels perform after it is over.

5. The best laxative foods after a fast are fresh sweet fruits; best of all are cherries and grapes, then a little soaked or stewed prunes. These fruits *must not be used after a meat-eater's first fast*, but only for people who have lived for a certain time on mucusless or at least mucus-poor foods—the "transition diet."

6. In the average case it is advisable to break the fast with raw and cooked starchless vegetables; stewed spinach has a specially good effect.

7. If the first meal foods do not cause any unpleasantness, you may eat as much as you can. Eating only a small quantity of food for the first 2 or 3 days without experiencing a bowel movement—owing to the small amount of food taken (another wrong advice given by "experts")—is dangerous.

8. If you are in the proper condition so that you can start eating with fruits, and you have no bowel movement after about an hour, then eat more or eat a vegetable meal as suggested above, eat until you bring out the waste accumulated during the fast with your stool, after eating the first meal.

Rules During the Fast

1. Clean the lower intestines as well as you can with enemas, at least every other day.

2. Before starting a longer fast, take a laxative occasionally, and by all means the day before you start the fast.

3. If possible, *remain in the fresh air*, day and night.

4. Take a walk, exercise, or some other physical work *only when you feel strong enough to do it;* if tired and weak, rest and sleep as much as you can.

5. On days that you feel weak, and you will experience such days when the waste is in the circulation, you will find that your sleep is restless and disturbed, and you may experience bad dreams. This is caused thru the poisons passing thru the brain. Doubt, loss of faith, will arise in your mind; then take this lesson and read it over and over, as well as the other fasting chapters and especially Lesson 5. Don't forget that you are, parenthetically speaking, lying on Nature's operating table; the most wonderful of all operations that could be performed; and without the use of a knife! If any extraordinary sensation occurs due to the drugs that are now in the circulation, *take an enema at once*, lie down, and if necessary break the fast, *but not with fruits.*

6. Whenever you arise after lying down, do it slowly, otherwise you may become dizzy. The latter condition is not serious, but you had better avoid it in this manner. It caused me considerable fear in the beginning, and I know a number of fasters and strict eaters who gave up when they experienced this sensation—lost their faith forever.

Fasting Drinks

The "fanatic" fasting enthusiast drinks only water. He thinks it best to avoid any trace of food whatsoever. I consider a light lemonade with a little honey or brown sugar or a fruit juice the best. Drink as often as you care to during the day, but in general not more than 2 or 3 quarts a day. The less you drink the more aggressive the fast works.

As a change, vegetable juices made from cooked starchless vegetables is very good during a longer fast. Raw tomato juice, etc., is also good. But if fruit juice—for example, orange juice, is used during a longer fast, be extremely careful because the fruit juices may cause the poisons to become loosened too rapidly without causing a bowel movement. I know a number of such fruit or fruit-juice fasts which failed completely because all mucus and all poisons if loosened too fast and too much at one time, disturbs all organs too greatly when in the circulation, and can be eliminated only thru the circulation and without the aid of bowel movements.

Morning Fast or Non-Breakfast Plan

The worst of all eating habits nowadays is to stuff the stomach with food early in the morning. In European countries, excepting England, no one takes a regular meal for breakfast; it is generally a drink of some kind with bread only.

The only time that man does not eat for 10 to 12 hours is during the night while he is asleep. As soon as his stomach is free from food, the body starts the eliminating process of a fast; therefore encumbered people awaken in the morning feeling miserable and usually have a heavily coated tongue. They have no appetite at all, yet they demand food, eat it, and feel better—WHY?

Another "Mystery" Revealed

This is one of the greatest problems I solved, and is one that puzzles all "experts" who believe it is the food itself. As soon as you refill the stomach with food, THE ELIMINATION IS STOPPED and you feel better! I must say that this secret which I discovered is undoubtedly the explanation of why eating became a habit and is no longer what Nature intended it should be, namely, a satisfaction, a compensation of Nature's need of food.

This habit of eating, affecting all civilized mankind and now physiologically explained, involves and proves the saying I coined long ago: "Life is a tragedy of nutrition." The more waste that man accumulates, the more he must eat to stop the elimination. I had patients who had to eat several times during the night to be able to sleep again. In other words, they had to put food in the stomach to avoid the digestion of mucus and poisons accumulated there!

FASTING (Part 4)

LESSON XX

You have just read in Lesson 19 about patients eating several times during the night in order to sleep again. You have been taught why this happens. Upon awakening you may perhaps feel fine, but instead of getting up you remain in bed and fall asleep again, have a bad dream, and actually feel miserable upon awakening the second time. You can now understand the exact reason for this.

As soon as you get up, move around, walk or exercise, the body is in an entirely different condition than during the sleep. The elimination is slowed down, the energy being used elsewhere.

If eating breakfast is eliminated from your daily menus, you will probably experience some harmless sensations, such as headaches for the first one or two days, but after that you will feel much better, work better, and enjoy your luncheon better than ever. Hundreds of severe cases have been cured by the "non-breakfast-fast" alone, without important changes in diet; proving that the habit of a full breakfast meal is the worst of all, and most injurious.

It is advisable and really of great advantage to allow the patient to have the same drink for breakfast that he is accustomed to; if he craves

132

coffee, let him continue his drink of coffee, but *absolutely* no SOLID food! Later on, replace the coffee with a warm vegetable juice, and still later change to lemonade. This change should be made gradually for the average mixed eater.

The 24-Hour Fast, or One Meal a Day Plan

As with the breakfast-fast, you can heal more severe cases with the 24-hour fast, or in cases of deep chronic encumbrance and drugs it is a careful, preliminary step to the necessary longer fasts. The best time to eat is in the afternoon, say, 3 or 4 o'clock P.M.

If the patient is on the mucusless or transition diet, let him eat the fruits first (fruits should always be eaten first), and after an elapse of 15 or 20 minutes eat the vegetables; but all should be eaten within an hour so that it is, so to say, one meal.

Fasting When Used in Connection with the Mucusless Diet Healing System

As I have stated before, I am no longer in favor of long fasts. In fact it may become criminal to let a patient fast for 30 or 40 days on water—contracting the avenues of circulation, which are continually filled up more and more with mucus and by dangerous old drugs and poisons, and at the same time rotten blood from his old "stock"; in fact actually starving from necessary vital food elements. No one can stand a fast of that kind without disadvantage, or without harming his vitality.

If fasting is to be used at all, then start at first
with the non-breakfast plan; then follow with the
24-hour fast for a while; then gradually increase up
to 3, 4 or 5-day fasts, eating between fasts for 1, 2,
3 or 4 days a mucusless diet, combined individually
as an elminiation adjustment, and at the same time
supplying and rebuilding the body continually with
and by the best elements contained in and found
only in mucusless foods.

Thru such an intermittent fast the blood is
gradually improved, regenerated, can more easily
stand the poisons and waste, and is able at the
same time to dissolve and eliminate "disease deposits" from the deepest tissues of the body; deposits
that no doctor ever dreamed existed, and that no
other method of healing has ever discovered or can
ever remove.

This, then, is the Mucusless Diet Healing System,
with fasting an essential part of it.

Fasting in Cases of Acute Disease

"Hunger Cures—Wonder Cures" was the title of
the first fasting book I ever read. It gave the
experiences of a country doctor, in which he said,
"No feverish, acute disease must nor can end with
death if Nature's instinctive command, to stop
eating thru lack of appetite, is followed."

It is insanity to give food to a pneumonia patient
with a high fever, for instance. Having had an
unusual contraction of the lung tissues by a
"cold," the pressed-out mucus goes into the circulation and produces an unusual heat-fever. The
human engine, already at the bursting point thru
heat, becomes more heated thru partaking of solid

food, meat broth, etc. (good, nourishing foods, so-called).

Air baths taken in the room, enemas, laxatives, cool lemonade would save the lives of thousands of young men who are now daily permitted to die, the innocent victims of pneumonia or other acute diseases—due to the stubborn ignorance of doctors and so-called highly civilized people.

The Superior Fast

Please try and memorize the lesson on Metabolism (Lesson 9) because it is the most important truth of my new physiology; also Lesson 5, and you will clearly understand fasting with all its possible sensations.

All experts, excepting myself, believe that you live from your own flesh during a fast. You know now that what they call Metabolism—"Metabolize your own flesh when you fast," is simply the elimination of waste.

The Indian "fakir," the greatest faster in the world today, is nothing but skin and bones. I learned that the cleaner you are, the easier it is to fast, and the longer you can stand it. In other words, in a body free from all waste and poisons, and when no solid foods are taken, the human body functions for the first time in its life without obstructions. The elasticity of the entire tissue system, and of the internal organs, especially of the spongy lungs, work with an entirely different vibration and efficiency than ever before, by air alone and without the slightest obstruction. Stated differently: "V" equals "P" and if you simply supply the "engine" with the necessary water which is used up, you ascend into a higher state of physical, mental and spiritual conditions. I call that the "Superior Fast."

If your blood "stock" is formed from eating the foods I teach, your brain will function in a manner that will surprise you. Your former life will take on the appearance of a dream, and for the first time in your existence your consciousness awakens to a real-self-consciousness.

Your mind, your thinking, your ideals, your aspirations and your philosophy changes fundamentally in such a way as to beggar description.

Your soul will shout for joy and triumph over all misery of life, leaving it all behind you. For the first time you will feel a vibration of vitality through your body (like a slight electric current) that shakes you delightfully.

You will learn and realize that fasting and superior fasting (and not volumes of psychology and philosophy) is the real and only key to a superior life; to the revelation of a superior world, and to the spiritual world.

"DESTRUCTIVE DIET OF CIVILIZATION AND THE MUCUSLESS DIET, THE NATURAL FOOD OF MAN"

LESSON XXI

You have now learned that total abstinence from food—FASTING—is the best and *most effective method* of healing. This proves with logical consequence how small a quantity is in fact necessary to sustain life and justifies my oft-repeated statement, "The wonder is that we live *in spite* of our excessive eating, in spite of our eating such wrong, destructive foods." In this light of truth it almost appears ridiculous to note the endless fight and confusion regarding dietetics, protein, mineral salts, vitamines, etc. The potential food value is not the first question at all. You cannot heal drunkenness by water without stopping the intake of alcohol. You cannot heal disease thru any kind of adjustments, treatments or diets, without stopping the eating of the foods which produce disease, the latter being 90% of the present day destructive diet of civilization.

I named the natural food of man, fruits and starchless greenleaf vegetables (as it is said in Genesis, "fruits and herbs") "Mucusless Diet," because mucus is the main and important and significant substance, while the other, wrong foods, contain, produce and encumber the human body with the matter of disease.

The entire "trash" of scientific dietetics, food values, statistics, etc., are useless and in vain as long as the first step is not taken, and that is to see the foods and their value from a principally different angle:

1. How far and how much they produce and leave disease matter (mucus) in the body.

2. Their dissolving, eliminating, healing properties. For this purpose I give you a special critique of the different foods, wrong foods especially, and you can see at once why they are "destructive" with no positive food value at all, but producing and leaving stored up waste in the body. See Lesson 14 and you will find that Berg's investigations proved to be the same that I found by intuition, experimenting and thru experience with myself and some thousands of patients.

MEATS

All are in a decomposing state, producing cadaver poisons, uric acid in the body and mucus; fats are the worst, even butter is unusable for the human body. No animals eat fat.

EGGS

Eggs are even worse than meats, because not only have eggs too high protein qualities, but they contain a gluey property much worse than meat and are therefore very constipating, quite more so than meat. Hard boiled eggs are less harmful, because the gluey qualities are destroyed; the white of eggs makes a very perfect glue.

MILK

Also makes a good glue for painting. Cow's milk is too rich for adults and for babies, and plainly destructive. A baby's stomach cannot digest what a calf can. If milk must be used then add at least half water and some milk sugar. Sour milk and buttermilk are less harmful and possess some laxative qualities; the gluey sticky properties disappear. Cottage cheese with stewed fruit (see Lesson 15) is good for transition diet. All other kinds of cheese are highly acid and are mucus formers.

FATS

All fats are acid forming, even those of vegetable origin, and are not used by the body. You will like, crave and use them only as long as you can still see mucus in the "magic mirror." What doctors call heat calories is caused by the fats in friction, obstruction in the circulation; they constipate the small blood vessels.

CEREALS

Cereals and all flour products form mucus and acid. The worst of all is white flour, because it makes the best paste. Bran, graham, whole wheat or rye bread are less harmful, because they have lost their sticky properties. When well done or toasted and well baked they are much less harmful. Raw cereals, if toasted, are to some extent a mucus broom, but contain stimulants, wrongly believed to be "food value." Pies made of rough unbaked dough are, according to my belief, absurd. When eaten with sweets and acids they are mucus and gas producers the same as French pastry.

LEGUMES

Lentils, dried beans and dried peas are too rich in protein, the same as meat and eggs. The peanut is a legume also.

POTATOES

A little better than flour products, because they contain more mineral salts (see Berg's tables), nor do they make a good, sticky paste. Sweet potatoes come close to natural sweets, but are too rich. Well fried, or crusty, baked like Saratoga chips, but without the animal grease, sweet potatoes are almost mucusless.

RICE

Is one of the greatest mucus formers and makes an excellent paste. I firmly believe thru my experience with serious cases of sickness (awful boils, etc.) prevalent among one-sided rice eaters, that rice is the foundational cause of leprosy, that terrible pestilence.

NUTS ·

All nuts are too rich in protein and fat and should be eaten only in winter, and then only sparingly. Nuts should be chewed together with some dried sweet fruits or honey, never with juicy fruits, because water and fat do not mix.

With the possible exception of nuts, the above represent about all of the foods which have to be prepared in some manner for eating; in fact they are tasteless unless specially prepared. What civilized man calls good to eat, delicious taste, is absurd. If the tongue is clean from mucus, and the nose for the first time free from dirty filth, both then become in fact "magic mirrors," "revelation organs," we may call them, the bridge of the sixth sense, that is, to sense the truth. You lose all desire for, and in fact cannot stand these stimulating spices, especially table salt, any longer. All of these unnatural foods are extremely bitter, and in fact for a normal nose they possess an offensive odor. The sense organs of man are in a pathological state embodied in a "pus-like" mucus and waste the same as the entire system, and being in a partly decayed condition themselves, they find this half rotten food palatable.

Even then you would and could not eat fats or animal foods without the cook's "preparation," that is, the art to cover the real taste and odor by spices and dressings. In fact taste and small vibrations are so far changed from the normal natural, that the heavy meat eater does not like the wonderful odor of a ripe banana. He prefers "haut gout," a French word meaning "the smell of half-decayed meat."

No scientific food value tables will convince you of the truth. You must sense it with your cleansed organs, how wrongly you are fooled into believing that you nourish and build up health and efficiency by these foods which are in reality destructive, because they stimulate, or more truthfully, stop the elimination of your old waste until the day of reckoning comes, when you are "officially" sick.

Paradoxically but true, civilized men *starve* to death thru ten times too much overeating of wrong, destructive foods; the "sack" (stomach) of digestion is enlarged and sunken, prolapsed, which condition dislocates and interferes with the proper functioning of the other organs. Its gland and pores of the walls are totally constipated and its elasticity as well as that of the intestines, with its vital function almost paralyzed. The abdomen is an abnormally enlarged sack of fatty, watery, dislocated organs thru which half or even more of the decayed foods of civilization slide, fermenting more and more into feces such as no animal has, *and this is called digestion!*

"Natural Food of Man," is the title of a book by Hereward Carrington.

There are some others by European authors, who prove and show from every point of view that man has and must have lived in prehistoric times from unfired, natural foods, fruits and greenleaf vegetables; however, a great philosopher once said: "Whatever must be first proved is doubtful." Whoever does not see or sense the truth at once will never believe it, even if it is proven thousands of times and from every possible angle. Even experts of fruit diet and raw food advocates have doubts that the degenerated man of today can live the Paradisical life.

It took me a few years of continual testing and experimenting until I was thoroughly convinced in spite of the fact that I believed at once. Now memorize what I teach in Lesson 5 and in the lessons on the New Physiology. All others are on the wrong track, misled by the protein fad as well as thru ignorance of how it looks inside of the body, what disease is, etc., but especially obstructive to a recognition of the truth is the ignorance as to what happens in the body if you eat fruits, fast or live on a mucusless diet. This fact that the interpretation of all and every sensation, which becomes more and more strange and new, the more and deeper healing process goes on, is based on the Old Physiology, and is therefore and must be consequently wrong. It is and was the "stumbling block" in the enlightenment about drugless healing in the first place, and advanced dietetics in particular. The natural diet was never systemically taken up, especially in combination with fasting, based on the truth of my new but correct physiology. This is absolutely necessary to learn and to understand. If you believe and know unshakeably the truth of Lesson 5, as well as the other lessons bearing on this subject, you will never doubt any more that fruits alone, even of but one kind, not only heal but nourish perfectly the human body, eliminating entirely the possibility of disease.

All others, not knowing these new truths and not possessing the necessary knowledge contained only in the Mucusless Diet Healing System, can never secure a perfectly clean body and a complete healing as well as possess an understanding of every situation.

They will never believe in the divine perfectness of the "Bread of Heaven," as it is said "The Lord will punish them by blindness," spiritual blindness, meaning that doubt, losing faith and belief will return again and again as long as waste and old poisons are circulating thru the brain for elimination. You are saved from this tragical error, I hope.

The special qualities of fruits, greenleaf vegetables and their perfectness as human food is plainly shown in Berg's tables.

The more free you become from any kind of waste and poisons, the more you will sense, feel and believe this greatest of all truths: "That the Paradisical diet is not only sufficient but brings you higher and higher, into physical and mental conditions never before experienced."

SEX

LESSON XXII

Sex Diseases

Thru the knowledge received in past lessons, you now know and can realize more than any Naturopath that there is no principal difference between any one kind of disease or another.

In this particular case, however, we find an exception, but only in so far as the symptoms of syphilis are concerned. Venereal diseases can be healed by diet and fasting easily for the simple reason that the patient is generally young in years. The cure becomes more aggravated, made more difficult, if drugs have been used. This, of course, has unfortunately happened in almost every case.

The so-called, characteristic symptoms of any kind of syphilitic disease are due to drugs of one or several kinds.

Gonorrhea

Nothing is easier to heal than this "cold" or "catarrh" at the sex organ, if untouched by drugs or injections. Doctors must admit that this condition may exist *without actual sex intercourse*, and therefore the germ can hardly be blamed. Gonorrhea is simply an elimination thru this natural elimination organ. One-sided meat eaters are very susceptible to this disease. Should a society girl contract it, they call it Leucorrhea.

If drug injections are used for any continued length of time the mucus and pus are thrown back into the prostatic gland, bladder, etc. In case of the female the entire womb, uterus, becomes inflamed, producing all kinds of typical woman diseases.

I had hundreds of such cases where Naturopathy failed to heal. Only fasting and this diet can help.

Roseola or rose rash, a syphilitical eczema, characterized by its "ham-gray" shade, the gray shade of the whites of the eye, is due to saltpetre acid, silver oxide injections. This also is the cause if gonorrhea enters the bone. All three are called syphilitic symptoms. Mercury is to blame for the hard chancre, secondary and tertiary syphilis.

The so-called "syphilis" does not exist in the animal kingdom, or among uncivilized people. Drugs are to blame for these destructive diseases, together with the diet of civilization. Sexual excesses are, of course, also to be blamed, but knowing exactly what disease is, you may agree if I expose the "mystery" of this disease with one stroke, i.e., drugs and extreme meat diet of civilization are far more to blame than all sexual excesses together.

For a patient poisoned especially by mercury a very careful and long transition diet is necessary, a radical fruit diet or fast may become harmful, not thru itself but caused by the drugs when they are dissolved and are back in the blood stream for elimination.

This condition requires so careful a control of the elimination that under all circumstances an expert with previous experience is required.

The so-very-common disease of dislocation, or falling of the womb, can be healed and only by this diet, together with long fastings combined with short fasts and with a long preparative diet.

Prostatic gland inflammation, stricture, bladder disease, hundreds of these patients have I saved from the tortures of doctors. I have made cures even after Naturopathy had failed by natural methods of elimination thru a new and perfect blood composition resulting from a mucusless diet.

Sex Psychology

It is significant for our civilization that sexual intercourse is seen as an immoral act. It is yet in the shade of a mystery. From a natural moral standpoint, says a philosopher, an unclean man has no right to produce a new being. "You shall not only generate, but reproduce yourself," says that great thinker, Nietzsche.

The fact is that we are all, with a very few exceptions, the cause of stimulants instead of love vibrations exclusively. Procreation is the most holy and divine act and charged with the highest responsibility, especially on the part of the father. A germ with the slightest defect is a generation not forward but downward. In very old and in classic civilization "Sex" was a cult, a religion, and in every mystology, poetry of all civilized people love is the great, main and general subject with the conscious or unconscious goal to reproduce his kind.

The fact is proven by statistics that every family of the city's population dies out, disappears with the third or fourth generation. In other words, the "sins" of the fathers and of the mothers produce diseased children and children's children degenerating into death with the third generation. What are these "sins?" You shall "love thy neighbor," and you do, perhaps, but you kill your own child, partly at least before it is born. Latent disease is general and universal. Besides the statistical fact that over fifty per cent of all young men in large cities have gonorrhea and young women leucorrhea, how can a defective germ grow into a perfect being between a filthy, mostly constipated colon and an unclean bladder of a civilized mother? And one of the worst tragedies of ignorance is the expectant mother who eats twice as much decayed "cadavers" of animals killed years ago in the stock yards of Chicago, because she is advised to "*eat for two*"—herself and the growing embryo.

Natural Control of Sex

"Nothing above the truth!—confess your sins to your own heart." It is a blasphemic paradox, tragical (there is no word strong enough) condition to stimulate a function continually with enforcement ignorantly expecting thereby to grow healthy and happy, believing you can suppress or control this function by preaching morals.

Nature does not listen to you, but you must listen to Nature if you want to be happy. We are the product of stimulations and not of natural love vibrations which eventually leads to impotence.

The only way to heal impotence is thru fasting

and this diet. See Lesson 5. Sex is a part of vitality, it is even, so to say, the barometer of regeneration, rejuvenation, youth, health and happiness.

I have seen sterility of the female healed, and every patient who earnestly took up this system for any kind of disease "rejuvenated."

No one of western civilization knows what genuine "love vibrations" mean from a body with clean blood composed of such ingredients that produce electric currents and static electricity sent out and received by "wireless"—hair. See what I have to say about hair in my "Rational Fasting." The beard of man is a secondary sex organ. Beardless and hairless and bald makes for a "second-rate" sex quality in every respect. See Judges 16: 13-18.

If you could believe how easy it is to control sex by this diet you would soon quit your steaks and eggs.

Masturbation, night emissions, prostitution, etc., are all eliminated from the sex life of anyone living on a mucusless diet after their body has become clean and powerful.

That saving, keeping the germ (an idea of modern experts) will nourish man's brain (high protein substance) is absurd. Love is the greatest power and it is, if natural, the highest "invisible food" from the infinite for soul and body.

SEX (Part 2)

LESSON XXIII

Motherhood and Eugenics

Motherhood with mucusless diet, before, during and after pregnancy is the development towards the Madonna-like, holy purity principally different from the dangerous so-called "ordinary" childbirth, with its ever-present risk of life, known in our present civilization.

If the female body is perfectly clean thru this diet, the menstruation disappears. In scripture it is called by the significant word "purification," which it in fact is; clean—no longer polluted by the monthly flow of impure blood and other wastes. This is the ideal condition of an inside purity capable of the "immaculate conception." When seen in the light of this truth the entire "Madonna mystery" is easily understood.

Every one of my female patients reported their menses as becoming less and less, then a two- three and four months' intermission, and finally entirely disappearing, which latter condition was experienced by those who went thru a perfect cleansing process by this diet.

Headaches, toothache, vomiting, and all other so-called "diseases of pregnancy" disappear, and

150

painless childbirth, an ample sufficiency of very sweet milk, babies that never cry, babies who are very differently "clean," as compared with others, are the wonderful facts I have learned from every woman becoming a mother after having lived on this diet.

It is not advisable to start a radical change in diet during pregnancy, or while nursing; this should be done at least two or three months before conception.

"Eating for two," with a special diet is unnecessary if the body is clean. Modern babies are overfed, hence these dangerous childbirths. The only reasonable change is to increase the eating of natural sweets such as figs, raisins, dates, grapes, etc.

Feeding the Baby

If mother's mi'   ____ to be insufficient or bad, do not use plain cow's milk; it should be diluted with at least one-third to one-half water and sweetened with milk sugar or honey. Start feeding the baby as soon as possible a teaspoonful of good fruit juices (juice from stewed beets is also good), and honey diluted in water between meals. The baby's craving is sweet, and proves that fruit sugar is the "essence" of all dietetics.

What is considered a well-fed and healthy looking baby, of average normal weight, is in reality pounds of waste or decayed milk.

Whether the baby is sick or not, as soon as you commence feeding it fruit juices and stewed mash fruits, you will learn from the elimination that I am correct. The change must therefore be made very carefully. Babies and children must go thru the same cleansing, healing process as do adults. I believe that a baby well nursed by good mother's milk on this diet and without "special" protein foods will grow wonderfully, and after the weaning period is over could be raised on apples alone.

As stated before, if a change of this kind in the baby's diet is made, they must be healed first— whether sick or not—cleansed from the waste of their "latent disease." This is the point that everyone refuses to believe, realize or understand.

Natural sweets are necessary for the growing child for building a strong skeleton. Lime is also important. (See Berg's Tables.)

I learned thru the few examples that we had in Europe, that the character, the mind in general of the growing child, is greatly and beneficially influenced by this diet, with the progress of the purity of the body. The "troubles" of raising children from which you can be saved are enormous. No more children's disease!

Thousands of mothers, unconsciously thru overeating half kill their children before they are born. Here then is the only and correct way to fight infantile mortality. *There is no higher moral duty of any kind than to produce a perfect being.*

Eugenics of a Diseaseless, Superior Race

Using a plant as a comparison, "motherhood" can be said to respect the QUALITY of the soul; "fatherhood" represents the quality of the seed—of the germ.

A relatively poor, almost barren soil but a good quality of seed produces a fairly good plant, but a *defective* seed, even though planted in the best soil, NOTHING.

Breeders of animals, especially horse breeders, know that the quality of a thoroughbred father goes thru endless generations, even spanning over a chin of "indifferent" mothers. This is why inheritance of good and bad qualities (tuberculosis for instance) skips a whole generation.

As in every respect of life this problem is different also, and, of course, is different in the case of a clean body on natural diet. Medical doctors and Naturopaths alike will hardly believe at all in the new principles and arguments which I have brought out, and postulated in this work. They reason and figure with the facts and experiences of the filthy body living on the unnatural diet of civilization.

You cannot reason about colors with a man born blind. You cannot use the old arguments and the old physiology to gainsay my statements.

Until you have personally experienced on your own body the truth of my teachings, you will have to accept and believe the new ones.

Realize, please, what this means—SUPERIOR FASTINGS—as they were taken by the prophets of old.

During a period covering some decades, and even partly today, the science of eugenics believed in the necessity of outside breeding. They consider outside breeding an absolute necessity for animals and the human race based on the bad results which accrued from the inbreeding of humans.

It is nothing less than the problem of the future of the American Nation—mixing races or inbreeding? The Jewish race is the answer, the only example in existence that inbreeding is natural and perfect. Marriage of close relationship fails simply because we have degenerated too far, in comparison with the people of their ancestor Abraham. Outside breeding is a "stimulation" with an apparently good result, lasting only for one or two generations and then, in general, the family dies out.

The European royal family kept their genealogical tree clean, securing good results only as long as they did not live in modern luxury. The families of noblemen are rapidly disappearing because they fail to continue the generation of males. The luxurious diet of today instead of the old-fashioned simplicity of centuries ago is to blame. Former generations lived as farmers (a more natural life). Today they are the typical "high livers" in modern Sodoms; no wonder an expiring degeneration is the result!

Predetermination of Sex

What I will endeavor to show here is how to produce a genius, and this will prove at the same time that the predetermination of the sex is based on a higher principle than on the time of conception only.

Again and again, diet is everything; man is what he eats! Are not all geniuses, great men, inventors, the greatest artists of every kind, born of poor parentage!

Why did the birth of boy babies increase during the European war? They will become good and intelligent men. Restriction in diet and restriction in sexual intercourse, that is all! The cleaner the body of both parents, the less frequent the intercourse, the smaller the quantity of good food, the greater the love vibrations become, and with these conditions the better the chance for a genius, and that is always a boy. The most ideal example of this truth, and it is said to be an historical fact, is this:

During the black plague centuries ago, a number of young people took refuge together in a house in the neighborhood of Florence, Italy. For weeks they had nothing to eat and then, of course, only sparsely. They became married and generated the family of the Medici, which produced the greatest statesmen, artists and scientists of every kind known in the history of western civilization.

We know that vitality vibrates thru a waste-free body more perfectly than one encumbered with food, that is the superior fast with its indescribable conditions. Yet more difficult of description are love vibrations—when man ascends to a God-like being, as he must have been in prehistoric times on the divine diet. The magnetic sex emanations become so wonderful that love combined with gluttony appears as a crime.

For the young couple to fast on their wedding day is a Jewish religious custom, but it is only a remainder of a hygienic law of that great statesman Moses—to generate geniuses thru superior waves of love thru the infinite.

It is the principle by which the male stock, when living on "clean" food has the opportunity to generate a diseaseless, superior one.

Everyone who travels a little further upwards on the road towards the "paradise-like" conditions of man will soon sense this truth. Man was once a higher, superior kind of being, not a species of the

monkey family! We are only a shade of the original
man, caused thru our degeneration, but you may
yet experience what cannot be described, that this
kind of eugenics is the fundamental truth of
evolution into "Heaven on Earth!"

THE ENFORCEMENT OF ELIMINATION BY
PHYSICAL ADJUSTMENTS
EXERCISES, SUN BATHS, INTERNAL BATHS
AND BATHING
LESSON XXIV

As shown in previous lessons all physical treatments vibrate—shake—the tissues and thereby stimulate the circulation in one way or another for the purpose and with the result of loosening and eliminating "foreign matters," the cause of all diseases. The human body does this itself, in the most perfect way, as soon as you fast or as soon as your blood composition has been changed by natural diet.

Physical treatments and physical culture can therefore be combined with this diet and fasting to enforce and to hasten the elimination. However, I must advise that extreme care be taken not to exaggerate—especially on "bad" days—days of strong elimination. If you are tired and you feel bad, then rest and sleep just as much as you can. On the days that you feel "good" during a fast or strict diet, you may take some physical treatment also, such as exercise, baths, massage, deep breathing, etc.

The most natural exercises and by far the best, are walking, dancing and singing; the latter being the natural breathing exercise with the added advantage of loosening by chest vibrations. An excellent "exercise" and one that everybody knows, is hiking in the mountains, for when climbing hills you increase your breathing in the most natural way, better and more harmoniously than with any "system" of exercises.

The cleaner you become the more easily you will understand what I teach in Lesson 5—that air and the other ingredients of the forests are "food"—invisible food.

Both hands should be free when walking, so as to permit continually the natural movements.

Outdoor garden work is another natural exercise.

By taking the proper care of your body you will generate health. The following exercises are suggested for those who desire to keep physically fit. I must again remind you that air is more necessary to life than food. Proper breathing is therefore essential. *Do not exercise in a close, stuffy room.* Stand before an open window. Take a deep, full breath with each exercise. Inhale through nose and expel through mouth. Stand before a mirror while exercising, and admire the suppleness and graceful manner in which you perform each movement. Fall in love with yourself if no one else will. Keep the feet about 15 inches apart—stand erect and use muscular tension.

Exercise No. 1

Standing erect, hands to the side, clinch the fists tightly. Raise arms slowly as high above the head as possible, taking a deep breath. Relax and expel breath. Repeat five times.

Exercise No. 2

Extend arms level with chest. Grasp hands tightly and pull to right side, resisting with left hand. Then go thru same motion pulling to left side. Relax after each motion, expelling breath. Repeat each exercise five times.

Exercise No. 3

Grasp left hand firmly with the right in front of body. Resisting with the left hand lift with the right, using full strength while raising the arms high above head. Take deep breath on upward motion, and relax before expelling. Repeat with the right hand resisting with the left, five times each.

Exercise No. 4

Clasp hands above the head allowing them to rest on head. Bend to the right side, pulling hard, then to the left five times, then alternate first right and then left. Between each movement take deep breath and expel when relaxed. This exercise is especially good for stimulating the liver.

Exercise No. 5

Clasp hands in back of neck, holding all muscles tense. Twist to the right, then to the left five times. Now pull to the right and then to the left five times. Now pull to the left and then to the right five times. Hold leg rigid, but permit body to sway.

Exercise No. 6

Grasp the hands behind the back and without bending the body raise arms up as far as possible. Inhale on upward motion, relax and expel. Repeat five times. This exercise is for developing the chest.

Exercise No. 7

Place right hand over right hip, clench left fist and raise left arm slowly, taking a deep breath. At the same time bend the body as far to the right as possible. Make it hurt. Relax and expel breath. Repeat with left hand placed on hip, and raising right arm with fist tightly clenched. Repeat each five times.

Exercise No. 8

Grasp hands firmly in front of breast, all muscles tense and twist to left. Now twist to right as far as possible. Do not permit feet to move. Inhale during motion, relax and expel breath. Repeat each exercise five times.

Exercise No. 9

Raise arms above the head as high as possible, and even permitting body to bend backwards. Now bend body forwards and without bending the knees try to touch the floor with your fingers. Exhale breath when relaxed. Repeat this exercise slowly five times, and gradually increase to 20 times.

Do not exhaust yourself in any of the exercises.

If the exercises make you stiff at first it is a sure sign that you needed them, and that they are doing you good. The soreness will soon wear off if you continue the exercises persistently. You may add other exercises to these, but be sure they have the deep breathing. *Play your phonograph when exercising.* Any snappy march piece will do. The vibrations from the music are wonderful. It is preferable to exercise the first thing in the morning—immediately upon arising. If clothing is worn it should be loose. Start with a few at first and gradually increase, but above all things, do not consider it a duty, but *put fun into them.* Dancing by yourself and bending movements to the accompaniment of music will prove very beneficial.

Sun Baths

Whenever you have an opportunity of doing so, take a sun bath. In the beginning do not exceed 20 to 30 minutes and keep the head covered. On "bad" days—days of great elimination—stay cool.

The cleaner you become the more you will enjoy the sun bath and the longer you will remain. You will also find that you can stand it much warmer. A short cool shower bath or a cool rub with a towel dampened in cold water immediately after the sun bath is good.

The sun bath is an excellent "invisible" waste eliminator, and rejuvenates the skin, causing it to become like silk and coloring it a natural brown. Civilized men of our race show by their white skin that they are sick from birth on; they inherit the mucused, white blood corpuscles—the "sign of death."

As all of the clothing should be removed during a sun bath, a small enclosure just long enough to lay in should be built in your back yard, or even on the roof, away from prying, inquisitive eyes. The clothing of civilization has made it impossible for man to secure his proper quota of the life-giving power of fresh air and sunshine, so essential to health and happiness. The direct rays of the sun on the naked body supply the electricity, energy and vitality to the human storage battery, renewing it in vigor, strength and virility.

Internal Baths

During the transition period, even though you have regular bowel movements, *it is advisable to wash out the lower colon.* The sticky waste, slimy mucus and various poisons which Nature is attempting to eject should be helped along as much as possible. A small bulb infant syringe can be used after the regular bowel movement, but for a thorough cleansing from two to three quarts of water should be used.

Try to have a natural bowel movement before injecting the water. The body should be in a reclining position, lying on the right side. The syringe must not be higher than three or four feet above patient. Water should be warm, not hot, and can be tested on your elbow. Should any discomfort be felt, stop the flow until the discomfort passes as the entire two or three quarts should be retained at one time. If the cramp or pain becomes too great, allow the water to pass from the colon and repeat the operation.

The water should remain in the intestines about

15 or 20 minutes, or as long as convenient. While still lying on your side gently massage the ascending colon in an upward motion. Then lie on the back with the knees drawn up and massage from right side of body to left; now turn over, lying on the left side and massage the left side with a downward motion. You should now be ready for ejecting the water. The best time to take an enema is just before retiring.

Bathing

Authorities differ on bathing almost as widely as they do on diet. The Mucusless Diet System will produce the "skin you love to touch" thru clean blood supply, and without the aid of cosmetics, lotions and cold creams.

It is not necessary to take a daily hot bath with soap and brush under ordinary conditions.

The morning "cold shower" during the entire year without any consideration of weather conditions is also inadvisable. There is no need to deliberately subject the body to an extreme shock, and in a number of cases more harm than good may result.

Needless to state the skin must be kept clean so that the pores may be permitted to properly function, and this can be accomplished by the following method: Place a basin of cool water before you. Dip the hands in basin and starting with the face rub briskly; wet the hands again and apply to the neck and shoulders; next rub the chest and stomach; next the arms and then the back, and last the legs and feet. Put the feet right into the basin if you care to. Keep moistening the hands as needed, but there is no necessity for throwing any quantity of water on the body. To dry off rub with the bare hands for five minutes if possible, until the body is all aglow or wipe with towel. This should be done upon arising immediately after you have taken your exercises. The results will surprise you. If you prefer a tub bath then allow about one inch of cold water to run into the tub. Sit in same with knees drawn up, and follow same rule of rubbing and massage as outlined above.

Remember that the air bath is just as essential as the water bath. A few minutes each day spent before an open window, upon arising and just before retiring, when all clothes are removed, massaging the body—helps the skin to retain its natural functioning qualities.

Always bear in mind that extremes of any kind are harmful. This applies to exercise, bathing and sleeping, as well as extremes in eating. Even extreme joy and happiness has been known to kill just as readily as extreme anger, hate and worry. Therefore, AVOID EXTREMES OF ALL KINDS.

A MESSAGE TO EHRETISTS

LESSON XXV

Dear Friends:

After careful and intelligent study of the foregoing lessons, you now know that disease consists of an unknown, decayed and fermented mass of matter in the human body, decades old—especially in the intestines and colon. You likewise know how unwise and ignorant it is to think that knowing what to eat is, alone, a complete diet of healing.

None of the recognized authorities know the tremendous importance of a thorough and deep cleansing of the human "cesspool." All are more or less "fooled" by Nature when they advise eating of fruits, with stomach and intestines clogged up by mucus and decomposed protein foods, eaten from childhood on.

You have been taught the result: should these poisons—cyanide of potassium—be dissolved too rapidly and permitted to enter the circulation, severe sensations—even death—may occur, and man's natural food; oranges, grapes, dates, etc., are blamed!

My teachings clearly prove that this hitherto unexplained ignorance regarding fruit diet is the "stumbling-block" for all other food research ex-

perts, who have made personal experimental tests.
Thousands of times have I heard the same cry—
even from young and supposedly healthy persons—"I became weak!" And all experts with the
exception of myself say, "Yes, you require more
protein; at least eat nuts."

During my personal tests, involving this same
problem, I tried to overcome this "stumbling-
block" hundreds of times. After a two-years' cure,
in Italy, of Bright's disease with consumptive tendency, by fasting and strict living on a mucus-less
diet, I ate two pounds of the sweetest grapes and
drank half a gallon of fresh, sweet grape juice,
made from the best and most wonderful grapes
grown there. Almost immediately I felt as though I
were going to die! A terrible sensation overcame
me, palpitation of the heart, extreme dizziness
which forced me to lie down, and I was seized with
severe pains in the stomach and intestines. After
ten minutes the great event occurred—a mucus
foaming diarrhea and vomiting of grape juice
mixed with acid-smelling mucus, and then the
greatest event of all! I felt so wonderfully well and
strong that I at once performed the knee-bending
and arm-stretching exercises 326 times con-
secutively. All obstructions had been removed!

For the first time in history I have shown what
man was when he lived without "fired" foods—during the pre-historic times (called Paradise) eating
fruits, the "bread of heaven."

For the first time in human history this "demon"
in the tragedy of human life has been shown—and
how he *can and must* be eliminated—before man
can again ascend to a Paradisical health, happiness,
immunity from disease and "God-like" being.

If the Garden of Eden—heaven on earth—ever existed it must have been a "fruit orchard." For thousands of years, through a wrong civilization, man has been tricked into unconscious suicide, reduced to slavery, to produce wrong food, "earning his bread by the sweat of his brow." Unnatural foods cause sickness and death.

"Peace on Earth" happiness and righteousness as yet remain a foolish dream. During thousands of years, God, Paradise, Heaven—Sin, Devil, Hell—seldom found an interpretation that a clear, reasoning mind would willingly accept. The average unfortunate fellowman thinks of God as a good and forgiving Father who will allow him to enter Paradise in another world—unpunished for any violations of His laws in Nature.

I have proven for the first time in history that the diet of Paradise is not only possible—good enough for a degenerate mankind, such as we now are—but that it is the Unconditional Necessity and the first step to real salvation and redemption from the misery of life. That it is a needed key to the lost paradise where disease, worry and sorrow—hate, fight and murder were unknown, and where there was no death, from unnatural causes at least.

"Man is what he eats" is a philosopher's greatest and truest statement.

You must now see why civilization, all religion, all philosophy, with their tremendous sacrifice of work, time, money, energy, is and has been part guesswork. The magic formula for "Heaven on Earth"—of the Paradise—must read like this:

"Eat your way into Paradise physically." But you cannot pass the gate, watched over by the angel with the flaming sword, until you have gone through the purgatory (cleansing fire) of fasting and diet of healing—a cleansing, a physiological purifying, by the "Flame of Life" in your own body! During thousands of years no one has escaped the struggle of death caused by an unnatural life, and *you* will have to face it some day.

But you, I and others who have learned this greatest and most important truth of life, are the only ones in existence today who are in fact, and not by mind only, out of the road of darkness and unconscious suicide, and into the light of the new civilization—the light of a physical regeneration—as the Foundation of Mental and Spiritual Revelation-like Progress to the light of a superior, that is to say, a spiritual world.

This will give an outline of the serious nature of my work—and the necessity for your help in carrying it through as the greatest deed you can perform—upon which depends not only your future destiny, but that of a suffering, unhappy mankind—on the verge of a physical and mental collapse.

ARNOLD EHRET.